IMPLANT PROSTHODONTICS

Clinical and Laboratory Procedures

SECOND EDITION

IMPLANT PROSTHODONTICS
Clinical and Laboratory Procedures

Patrick J. Stevens, DDS
Private Practice, Prosthodontics
Spokane, Washington

Edward J. Fredrickson, DDS, FICD
Private Practice, Prosthodontics
Spokane, Washington

Maurice L. Gress, CDT, FNBC
President, AU Dental Ceramics, Inc.
Spokane, Washington

with 757 illustrations, including 709 in color

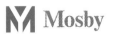 Mosby

St. Louis Baltimore Boston Carlsbad Chicago Minneapolis New York Philadelphia Portland
London Milan Sydney Tokyo Toronto

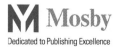

Mosby
Dedicated to Publishing Excellence

Editor-in-Chief: **John Schrefer**
Editor: **Penny Rudolph**
Developmental Editor: **Kimberly Frare**
Project Manager: **Dana Peick**
Senior Production Editor: **Jeffrey Patterson**
Designer: **Amy Buxton**

SECOND EDITION

Mosby, Inc.
A Harcourt Health Sciences Company
11830 Westline Industrial Drive
St. Louis, Missouri 64146

Printed in the United States of America

International Standard Book Number 0-8151-3567-X

00 01 02 03 04 AC/KPT 9 8 7 6 5 4 3 2 1

CONTRIBUTORS

Neal D. Futran, MD, DMD
Assistant Professor
Department of Otolaryngology
Head and Neck Surgery
University of Washington
Seattle, Washington

Abraham Ingber, DDS
Adjunct Assistant Clinical Professor
Department of Restorative Sciences/Biomaterials
Boston University
School of Dental Medicine
Boston, Massachusetts

Joseph Kravitz, DDS, MS
Clinical Instructor
Department of Restorative Dentistry,
Postgraduate Prosthodontics
University of Maryland Dental School
Baltimore, Maryland

Brien R. Lang, DDS, MS
Professor Emeritus
Department of BMS/Prosthodontics
University of Michigan
School of Dentistry

Steven G. Lewis, DMD
Director, Implant Prosthodontics
Division of Oral and Maxillofacial Surgery
University of Cincinnatti
Cincinnatti, Ohio

Gayle S. Orton, RDH, MEd
Professor
Department of Dental Hygiene
Eastern Washington University
Cheney, Washington

Vincent Prestipino, DDS
Assistant Clinical Professor
Postgraduate Prosthodontics,
Department of Restorative Dentistry
University of Maryland Dental School
Baltimore, Maryland

David L. Reimers, CDT
Edgewood Dental Laboratory, Inc.
Mukilteo, Washington

Jeffrey E. Rubenstein, DMD, MS
Associate Professor
Department of Prosthodontics
University of Washington
School of Dentistry
Seattle, Washington

Robert K. Steadman, DDS
Diplomate
American Board of Oral and Maxillofacial Surgery
Fellow
AAOMS, IAOMS, AACS, ACOMS
Spokane, Washington

Deborah L. Steele, RDH, BS
Department of Maxillofacial Prosthodontics
L.K.Nakayama, DDS
Beaverton, Oregon

Clark O. Taylor, MS, DDS
Director
Institute of Facial Surgery
Missoula, Montana and Bismarck, North Dakota;
Associate Professor of Surgery
Department of Surgery
University of Nebraska
Omaha, Nebraska

Philip Worthington, MD, DDS, BSc, FDSRCS
Professor and Chairman
Department of Oral and Maxillofacial Surgery
University of Washington
School of Dentistry
Seattle, Washington

DEDICATION

The scientific method is defined in the fourth edition of Blakiston's Gould Medical Dictionary as "The principles and procedures of science which seeks to establish knowledge systematically and objectively, and therefore, requires the recognition of a phenomenon or problem, the accumulation of pertinent data through observation and experimentation, the formation of a hypothesis to explain the phenomenon, and the testing and confirmation of the hypothesis based on the accumulated data."

The Hippocratic oath written by Hippocrates (Greek physician 460-377 BC) in part states, "I will follow that system of regimen which, according to my ability and judgment, I consider for the benefit of my patients, and abstain from whatever is deleterious and mischievous…with purity and holiness I will pass my life and practice my art."

Professor Per-Ingvar Branemark, Professor, M.D., Ph.D., O.Phc., as a scientist and physician, has adhered to these methods and oaths while changing the lives of patients, physicians, and dentists. The authors would like to acknowledge Professor Branemark for his contribution to dentistry as well as the betterment of mankind.

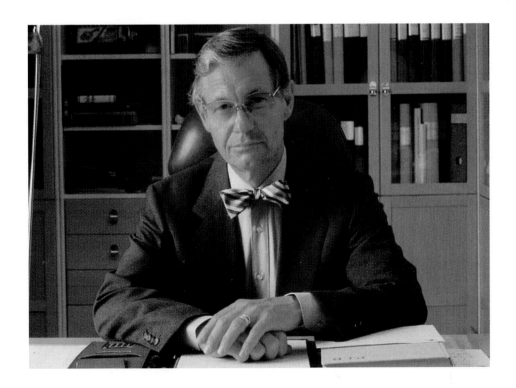

PREFACE

The rehabilitation of patients with failing or missing dentition using titanium implants has been dramatically changed since Professor Per-Ingvar Branemark set out to train select teams of surgeons and prosthodontists in the early 1980s. The early North American pioneers included teams in Toronto, Canada, followed by groups in New York; Washington, D.C.; Spokane, Washington; and Seattle, Washington. Basic training courses provided by the original teams have trained thousands of dentists in surgical and prosthetic techniques. Most dental schools now include courses in teaching undergraduate students introductory science and techniques involving dental implants. Surgical training has become a most important component in the curriculum of dental specialty training for oral and maxillofacial surgery and periodontics. Postdoctoral prosthodontic education has responded to the demands of implant rehabilitation with an extra year devoted to implant prosthodontics. Special fellowships are available limited to implant prosthetics.

This extra curriculum is necessary to provide basic skills and knowledge to plan and complete simple to more complex implant therapy. Even with postdoctoral training, the most complex implant rehabilitations are perhaps beyond the skill level of most specialists right out of training programs. There is no replacement for experience and developing advanced skills by completing more basic techniques well before tackling the most complex rehabilitations. As with all skills, working toward perfection requires experience, continued training, and close collaboration with all members of the implant team.

A disturbing trend toward short-cutting the learning process is being led by certain dental implant manufacturers and dental laboratories. Two-day training courses are offered, which in some cases lead dentists to believe that the most complex full-mouth implant rehabilitation can be attempted with success. Dental laboratories offer services such as treatment planning and component selection and even provide typed estimates for presentations to patients. This can lead to disaster for patients and restorative dentists.

Patient treatment must be planned and undertaken only by those whose skill and experience match the patients' needs. Implant rehabilitation requires extensive knowledge of dental materials, radiographic interpretation, bone biology, anatomy, engineering, speech, and esthetics as well as many other areas of study. Current dental and medical research and statistics on implant-related complications, failures, and solutions to minimize these problems must be understood to prevent mistreatment of patients. The responsibility for patient treatment belongs solely to the restorative dentist and surgeon rendering treatment.

Advances in surgical and prosthetic techniques, as well as logarithmic growth in the number of available implant components has greatly complicated implant dentistry. Surgeons, prosthodontists, and restorative dentists who feel that an implant procedure is beyond their current level of experience should acquire advanced training or refer the patient to specialists with the experience to complete procedures safely.

Some dental laboratories and implant manufacturers are obviously interested only in profit and selling their products and services. They cannot replace the knowledge and experience gained by advanced training and years of clinical experience.

Implant manufacturers have gone as far as promoting techniques where the surgeon makes impressions of the dental implant at the time of implant placement, and the dental laboratory can then directly fabricate temporary and definite restorations while almost bypassing the prosthetic dentist altogether. This may lead to disaster unless the restorative dentist is involved from treatment planning, to directing implant position and prosthetic design, to overseeing laboratory proceedings and delivering the provisional and final prosthetics.

There is also a trend in implant prosthetics to produce cementable implant-supported prosthetics. Procedures for cementable prosthetics are proclaimed to be superior for a variety of reasons. The most common rationale is that dentists are familiar with crown and bridge procedures and therefore cementable implant prosthetics require less training and are easier. Composite resin covering access holes causing cosmetic compromise, to the absurd notion that the access holes preclude tripodized occlusion, have been mentioned as reasons to avoid screw-retained prosthetics.

Multiple-implant prosthetics that are cementable are in most cases not predictably retrievable even when placed with temporary cement. Tapping off cemented implant prosthetics can fracture porcelain, implant components, and possibly break implants themselves. The accumulative force of years of function and parafunction has proved to cause complications with screw-retained prosthetics, which will obviously happen with cement-retained prosthetics as well. The screw retained prosthesis is retrievable for component replacement, modification, and repair. The psychologic and financial trauma to patients is minimized when a retrievable prosthesis can be easily removed and repaired. The cementable prosthesis will often require cutting the superstructure, splitting crown units to break cement bonds, and may ultimately break implant components if improper force is applied. Full-arch prosthetics cost patients tens of thousands of dollars initially. Subsequent complications requiring destruction and remake of prosthetics is a great disservice to the patient bordering on malpractice, especially since a retrievable design can be fixed at a fraction of the cost. Remember, the patient's well-being is more important than a "simpler" technique.

Patrick J. Stevens, DDS

CONTENTS

Evolution of Implant Prosthetics

Loss of teeth, eventual edentulism, and the wearing of complete dentures have been part of the expected course of aging by the general population. The incidence of edentulism in the Western world has posed a challenge to prosthodontists and oral surgeons, encouraging them to devise acceptable prosthetic results for patients. Although the patient may adapt well to the complete denture prosthesis, the decrease in masticatory function, in comparison with that of complete natural dentition, has been well documented. Years of wearing complete dentures leads to progressive bone resorption. The resorptive process decreases surface area for prosthesis support, eliminates favorable anatomy for retention, and results in unfavorable denture-bearing areas. These results include unfavorably positioned muscle attachments, mental nerve sensitivity, and irregular bony configurations that underlie thin mucosa. Loss of lateral stability and retention increases prosthesis movement, resulting in increased friction and mucosal irritation.

Many surgical procedures have been developed over the years to restore more favorable anatomy for prosthesis support. Some of these include vestibuloplasty, vestibuloplasty with skin or mucosal grafting, and augmentation with either rib- or hipbone-grafting procedures. These procedures offered short-term improvement in denture stability and retention; however, none showed long-term clinical success. Implanting artificial material to aid in denture retention has been used for many years with varying degrees of clinical success. Scientific documentation through animal studies and clinical trials was lacking for most techniques.

The first scientifically based study on the biocompatibility of implantable materials began in Sweden in 1952. Animal studies, including work with rabbits and dogs, indicated that properly prepared surgical-grade titanium in combination with careful surgical technique resulted in a predictable biologic response and a phenomenon that was termed *osseointegration* by its progenitor, Professor Per-Ingvar Branemark of Göteborg, Sweden.

Branemark defines the osseointegration process in his book, *Tissue Integrated Prostheses: Osseointegration in Clinical Dentistry*, as the "direct structural and functional connection between ordered, living bone and the surface of a load-carrying implant. Creation and maintenance of osseointegration, therefore, depends on the understanding of the tissue's healing, repair, and remodeling capacities." The first edentulous patients were treated in Sweden with titanium implants in 1965. The long-term clinical success of the Swedes and other international teams who were following proper protocol is well documented.

The original clinical protocol in Sweden called for restoring edentulous mandibles with fixed prosthetics. These were the neediest patients from a functional standpoint and provided a large available patient population for research protocols, which began after animal studies were completed. Fewer upper jaws were restored as well using the same components. Early abutment design involved what is still known as the standard abutment placed on multiple implants. One-piece fixed prosthetics were attached to the abutments with gold alloy screws. Components were designed for function with little concern for esthetics. These same components were basically the only ones available commercially worldwide until 1987 to 1988.

As restorative dentists and surgeons attempted to restore many edentulous situations with implants, the limitations of the available components led to the development of prosthetic components that allow more esthetic restorations. Dental laboratory technicians, dentists, and implant companies began responding to esthetic desires of patients paying thousands of dollars for implant rehabilitation by developing components designed to restore smaller edentulous areas. Single-tooth restorations and smaller prostheses supported by two or three implants in partially edentulous areas showed the most complications with loosening components and broken screws and implants. Prosthetics were developed that bypassed the abutments and attached directly to the implant. This reduced the space needed for components and allowed porcelain to be placed at or below tissue level.

The complications documented in the first edition of this text were a result of components that were not large or strong enough for certain anatomic deficits. The design and torque specifications allowed connections between implants, abutments, and prosthetics to loosen and fracture, especially in one- to two-implant posterior restorations. As with all new designs, it may take years for problems to develop clinically. Implants placed in areas of extreme resorption and poor quality bone lead to unesthetic, biomechanically unsound prosthetics.

Unfavorable anatomic relationships resulting from mandibular and maxillary resorption patterns were often found to be better surgically corrected with bone grafting and orthognathic surgery to restore bony and soft-tissue contours to preextraction or ideal form before implants are placed. This leads to less stress on implants and prosthetic components while eliminating large cantilevers and restoring facial contours, allowing the most ideal esthetic matrix for prosthetic reconstruction.

Advances in surgical technique to establish this ideal matrix have occurred with the worldwide spread of implant rehabilitation. These surgical techniques require advanced treatment planning and cooperation between the different dental specialties. When natural dentition is present, endodontic, periodontal, and orthodontic evaluation and expertise are needed, as well as surgical and prosthetic impute. Ultimately the dental laboratory technician must be able to fabricate natural-looking functional prosthetics with an expectation that the work will last for decades. The original team concept discussed in the first edition remains essential.

Newer components have been developed that allow stronger joints between components; choices for restoring each anatomic situation are much more numerous than they were 10 years ago. Wider-diameter implants and larger-diameter screws with higher torque requirements have been developed in hope of reducing complications. Advances in dental materials, especially dental porcelain, have occurred. The computer age has led to possibilities that may alter the practice of dentistry greatly.

Advances in plastic surgery and microvascular grafting have allowed the head and neck cancer patient with large anatomic defects to have hope of normal function and improved esthetics. The use of dental implants as anchorage for prosthetics in maxillofacial defects has opened a new realm of rehabilitation with implants. Professor Branemark has used the knowledge gained from dental and maxillofacial rehabilitation with implants to perform orthopedic advances, including attaching artificial limbs. The evolution of implant prosthetics is impressive and expanding in logarithmic fashion. The ultimate goal is always to improve patients' lives in a safe and predictable way.

The increase in clinical applications of dental implants in conjunction with economically driven development of literally thousands of commercially available components has created potential problems. The techniques and components to restore each edentulous area are as numerous as the companies manufacturing and marketing the components. The education necessary to select the appropriate systems and techniques is often controlled by groups with economic interest in the particular components they promote. Long-term testing of all components to simulate 5 or more years of clinical use is a standard not being followed or regulated for most components. Patients and the dentist who is responsible for providing implant rehabilitation will be affected by the complications that arise from improperly tested components.

The authors of this text recommend that the dentists selecting components choose companies with a long track record with the components that they sell. Education available for general dentists and specialists can vary from 1- to 2-day courses to study clubs involving extensive hands-on education. Dental schools also have educational programs that cover very basic education for dentists beginning their implant education to advanced courses for the experienced implant surgeon and restorative dentist. The authors recommend that restorative dentists maximize their implant education using textbooks, refereed prosthodontic and implant journals, and an involvement in study clubs. The patient's safety and long-term success with implant-based restorative dentistry is paramount. Referral to experienced dental specialists is recommended for the most complicated situations if the restorative dentist is not experienced in a particular technique.

Treatment Planning and Component Selection

TREATMENT PLANNING

Implant placement, including position, angulation, and selection of appropriate length and width, is crucial for allowing esthetic, functional, and biomechanically sound implant prosthetics. Communication between the surgeon, restorative dentist, and laboratory technician is necessary to ensure proper fixture placement. Improper implant position and angulation is evident in Figs. 2-1 to 2-6. Correction of poor implant angulation may be accomplished with various angulated or custom abutments, but in many instances the poor position may interfere with speech, compromise esthetics, or violate the neutral zone (see Figs. 2-3 and 2-4). It is the authors' opinion that fixtures can no longer be placed just where the bone is but that bone grafting should be used in situations where fixture position otherwise would compromise the final prosthetics. *If the bone grafting is not done, the fixtures should not be placed in compromised positions.* Meetings between restorative dentists and surgeons using photographs, radiographs, and mounted diagnostic casts with trial tooth settings in place should occur in even the most straightforward-appearing situations to ensure ideal implant position.

Diagnostic and Surgical Templates

A diagnostic template incorporating stainless steel balls is used for treatment planning of the implant position. A panoramic radiograph is made with the template seated in the mouth to evaluate vertical bone height in relation to the mental foramen and inferior alveolar nerve in the mandible. Bone height in the maxilla below the nasal floor and maxillary sinus can be measured. The actual diameter and position of the stainless steel balls in the template relative to the diameter and the position measured on the radiograph help determine distortion of size and position as seen on the radiographs.

Several configurations can be used depending on the type of implant prosthesis that is planned. The ball bearings can be attached to the existing prosthesis with sticky wax before making the radiograph (Fig. 2-7). For single-tooth or partially edentulous situations where an existing prosthesis is absent, a custom diagnostic template is made from impressions and mounted study casts with diagnostic setups, which are processed in clear acrylic carried over the incisal edge of the remaining teeth (Figs. 2-8 to 2-11). Stainless steel balls are placed in the template at desired implant sites (Fig. 2-12). Radiographs are then made with templates positioned on the teeth (Figs. 2-13 and 2-14). Analysis of radiographs helps determine bone height for implant placement, and prosthetic options can be discussed with the patient. It is important that prosthetic options, as well as complications from anatomic structures, are understood by the patient. Documentation and signed consent forms prevent misunderstanding when the prosthesis is completed.

Surgical Template

After the treatment plan has been determined by the restorative dentist and surgeon, a surgical template is fabricated by the dental technician. The configuration of the template is determined by the type of prosthesis. The diagnostic stent, in most applications, may be altered for use in the implant surgery (Fig. 2-15). The alteration is accomplished by relieving the inferior border of the template 3 to 4 mm to allow the surgeon room for soft-tissue reflection.

If the diagnostic template is not available, diagnostic casts are mounted (Fig. 2-16). The most posterior sites for the implant placement are marked anterior to the mandibular mental foramen bilaterally (Fig. 2-17). These sites are identified, and reference marks are made on the cast. The anterior residual ridge between the reference points is blocked out between the labial and the lingual sulci using three layers of baseplate wax (Fig. 2-18). This relief area allows the surgical template to be completely seated on the posterior ridge and will not interfere with tissue reflection in the anterior area. An impression of the relief cast is made for ease of separation and duplicated in the laboratory plaster (Fig. 2-19). A vacuum-forming machine is used to adapt a single layer of 0.080 inch plastic sheet material over this duplicate cast (Fig. 2-20). The excess material is trimmed, and the borders are adjusted to the cast and finished in a similar procedure as a denture border. Guide-pin holes are drilled through the relief area for fixture placement by the restorative dentist (Fig. 2-21). The fit and implant position is checked on the mounted diagnostic cast before delivery to the oral surgeon (Fig. 2-22). Another method for producing a template is to take an impression of the existing prosthesis and duplicate it in methylmethacrylate resin (Fig. 2-23). Guide pins are placed indicating position and angulation of the implants

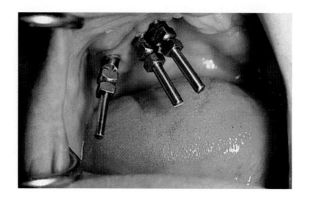

Figure 2-1

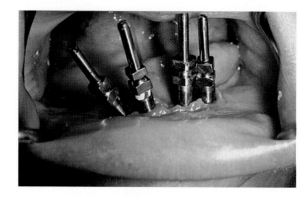

Figure 2-2

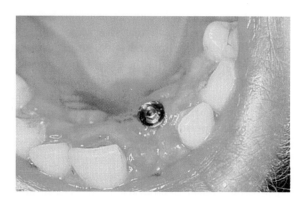

Figure 2-3

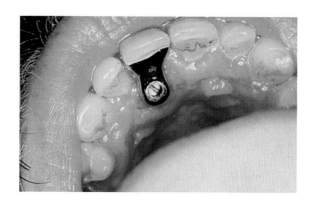

Figure 2-4

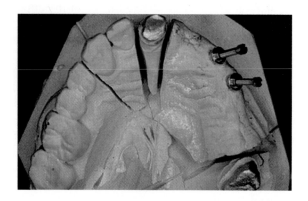

Figure 2-5

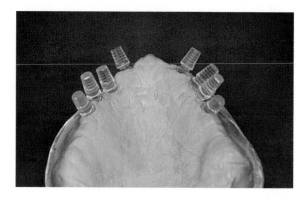

Figure 2-6

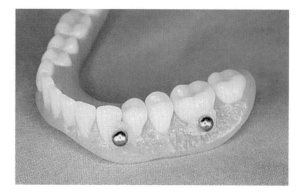

Figure 2-7

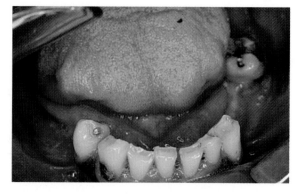

Figure 2-8

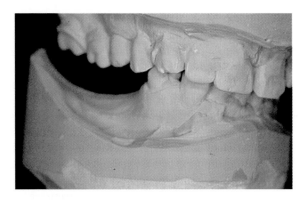

Figure 2-9

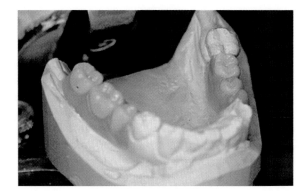

Figure 2-10

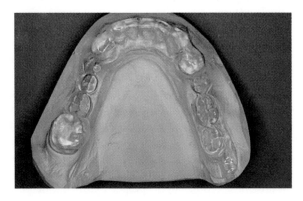

Figure 2-11

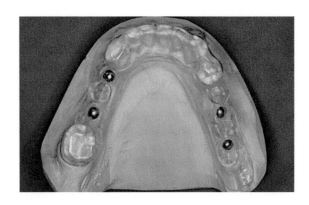

Figure 2-12

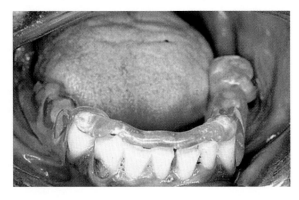

Figure 2-13

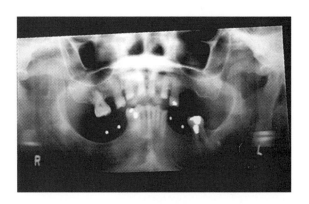

Figure 2-14

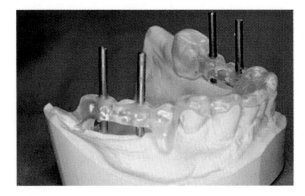

Figure 2-15

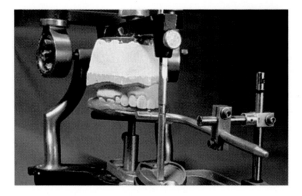

Figure 2-16

(Fig. 2-24). A duplicate of the existing maxillary denture and its relationship to the mandibular ridge are shown in Fig. 2-25.

Guide pins are placed to indicate position and angulation (Fig. 2-26). This method is unique because it does not interfere with the reflection of tissue during surgery. There are additional applications of the surgical template for the single-tooth prosthesis (Figs. 2-27 to 2-30), the anterior partially edentulous prosthesis (Figs. 2-31 to 2-34), and the posterior unilateral and bilateral partially edentulous prosthesis.

COMPONENT SELECTION
Implant Selection

This section discusses implant size appropriate for different areas of the mouth. The only factor affecting implant length is the height of bone available without encroachment on anatomic structures, such as the inferior alveolar nerve, maxillary sinus, and floor of the nose. Rarely, implant length may be limited by the root of an adjacent tooth. The longer the implant, the greater surface area available for integration. Long implants in the anterior mandible and the pterygomaxillary region (see Chapter 4) may be necessary to engage maximum cortical bone.

The implant diameter has a more critical effect on prosthetic design. Wider-diameter implants have greater surface area for integration and therefore may allow prosthetic support in areas where standard-diameter (3.75 mm) implants might fail. Specifically, wide-diameter implants (4.0, 5.0 mm) help compensate for poor bone quality and volume in the maxillary posterior as well as above the inferior alveolar nerve in the posterior mandible. Wide-diameter implants have thicker walls and resist the fracturing that has been reported with standard-diameter implants, supporting small-span prosthetics and single teeth in posterior restorations.

The other components designed for use only with the larger-diameter implants include wide-platform abutments and larger-diameter abutment and prosthetic screws. Chapter 9 describes prosthetic applications of wide-diameter components and the biomechanical reasons that complications are greatly reduced. Narrow-diameter implants are available for single anterior restorations specifically used for maxillary laterals and mandibular incisors where space between natural teeth is limited.

Abutment Selection

Many different abutments are available for different prosthetic applications. Implant position and angulation may require different abutments to allow optimum esthetics. Lack of intermaxillary space may preclude traditional abutments and require special or custom abutments. Visual inspection after abutment surgery may give an indication of appropriate abutment selection, but the proper abutment can only be

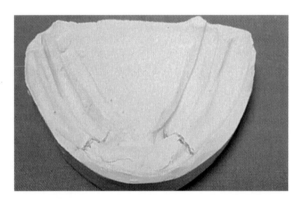

Figure 2-17

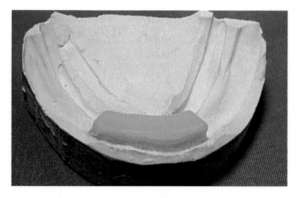

Figure 2-18

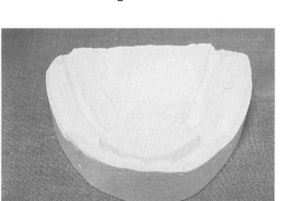

Figure 2-19

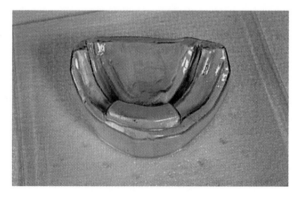

Figure 2-20

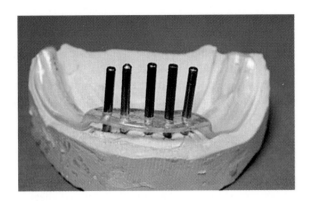

Figure 2-21

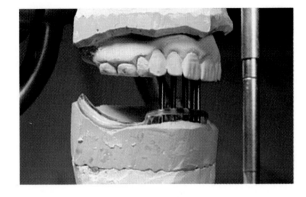

Figure 2-22

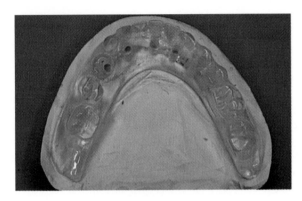

Figure 2-23

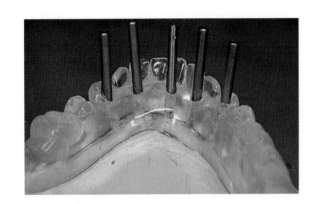

Figure 2-24

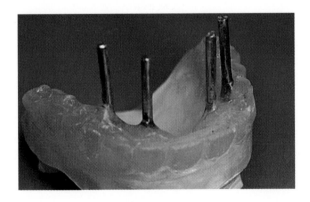

Figure 2-25

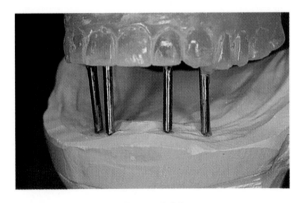

Figure 2-26

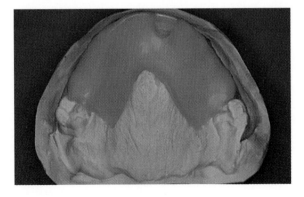

Figure 2-27

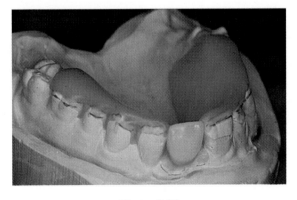

Figure 2-28

selected by diagnostic procedures including trial denture setups or provisional restorations on a diagnostic cast with abutments incorporated in the trial restoration. Abutments come in sterile packaging and are not to be used in more than one patient. Abutments cost up to $200 each; therefore mistakes in abutment selection can be time consuming and costly.

Aluminum abutment analogs are available for use in diagnostic procedures to select the proper abutments (Figs. 2-35 to 2-42). These trial abutments are inexpensive and reusable, thus allowing a precise method for determining correct abutments.

Procedure

Temporary healing abutments should be selected at the abutment operation for all situations where abutment type is not absolutely known. After adequate healing following abutment surgery, the healing abutments are removed using a hexagonal screwdriver. A cotton pellet slightly larger than the abutment diameter is placed with topical anesthetic into the tissue access after abutment removal. Single-tooth implant level impression copings are placed on each implant. Radiographs are made to confirm proper seating over the hexagonal head of the implant. The impression is made in the usual fashion. After impression removal, cotton pellets with

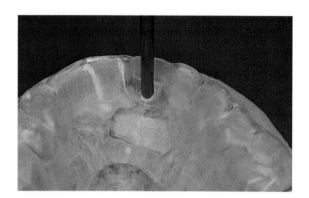

Figure 2-29

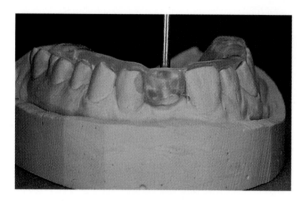

Figure 2-30

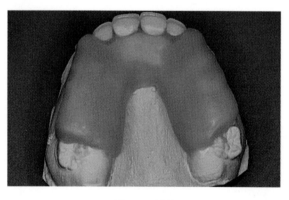

Figure 2-31

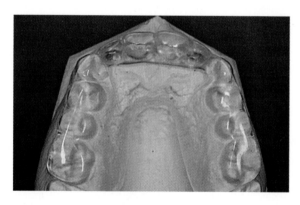

Figure 2-32

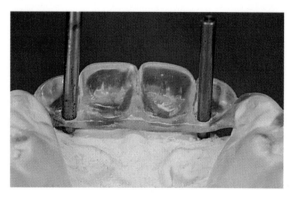

Figure 2-33

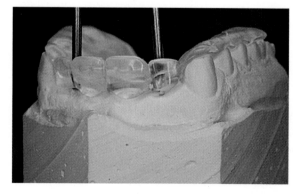

Figure 2-34

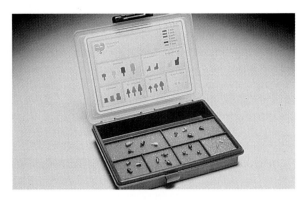

Figure 2-35

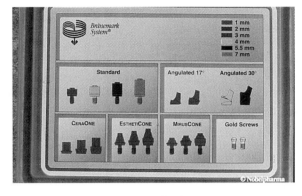

Figure 2-36

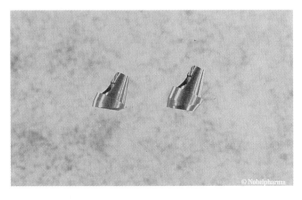

Figure 2-37

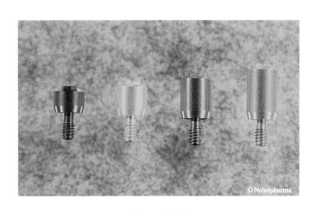

Figure 2-38

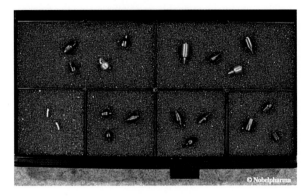

Figure 2-39

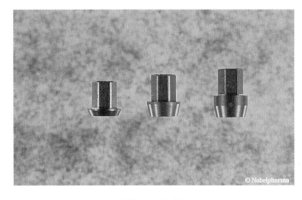

Figure 2-40

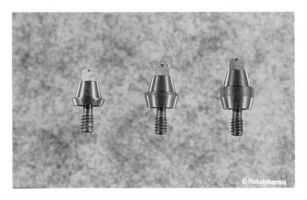

Figure 2-41

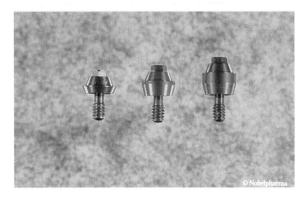

Figure 2-42

topical anesthetic are again placed to avoid tissue collapse and provide comfort while healing abutments are replaced.

Implant analogs are placed on the impression copings, and the impression is poured in die stone with a resilient material surrounding the abutments. The diagnostic cast is used with the trial denture setup to select trial abutments. Diagnostic wax-up can then be completed to evaluate abutments for metal display, proper angulation and position, and intermaxillary space limitations. Inappropriate abutments may be removed and replaced with other trial abutments until a diagnostic wax-up is completed, which allows for an ideal restoration.

Ideal implant position will allow the screw access hole to be positioned through the cingulum area of the anterior teeth and through the center of the occlusal surface of posterior teeth. Implants angled toward the buccal may compromise esthetics and restoration strength by having screw access holes that angle through the incisal edge or labial surface of the prosthesis. Fixtures angled lingually may extend the metal framework into the neutral zone and cause potential speech difficulties, making access for screw placement more difficult. Implants positioned or angled into interproximal areas may also compromise esthetics and hygiene. The additional time and expense of improper abutment selection followed by casting an inappropriate implant framework can be avoided by using the abutment selection kit for diagnostic workup before mistakes are made.

Rarely, the proper abutment may not be available to solve problems associated with poor implant placement. Proper presurgical planning involving communication between the surgeon, restorative dentist, laboratory technician, and use of surgical templates made from presurgical diagnostic procedures should eliminate problems in fabricating the final prosthesis. Custom titanium abutments and restorations can be designed and fabricated using computer-generated methods as described in Chapter 13.

Edentulous Mandible: Fixed Prosthetics

Most complaints about dentures are from patients who are completely edentulous on the mandibular arch. Resorption of the alveolar ridge results in decreased surface area and anatomic configuration, which lessens denture retention and stability. The increase in movement of the lower denture results in mucosal irritation and ulceration, reducing masticatory efficiency and increasing patient discomfort. As the mandibular resorptive process continues, the denture may impinge on the mental foramen and nerve and on the genial tubercles, which may hamper prosthesis use altogether.

When a patient first complains about the mandibular denture, a thorough evaluation of the existing prosthesis is made. This procedure includes an evaluation of the proper denture extensions, the dental occlusion, and the vertical dimension of the occlusion. The patient is given a head and neck evaluation, including a cancer screening, and radiographic and intraoral examinations are completed and charted. Health history questionnaires are administered and followed by an in-depth patient interview. The patient's denture history is charted to evaluate his or her expectations. The process of patient awareness and education is completed, informing the patient of the many prosthetic options. The patient's choices include having no treatment, relining an existing prosthesis, making a new prosthesis, or fabricating one of the various implant-supported prostheses. Different prosthetic options shown in the literature, on dental models, or in videotapes are helpful for patient education. If the patient is interested in pursuing an implant-supported prosthesis, a referral is made for surgical evaluation.

After the surgeon has evaluated the amount of bone the patient has available and the number of implants that can be predictably placed, a second consultation is scheduled to determine the best prosthetic option for the patient from functional, esthetic, hygienic, and financial standpoints. The patient's dexterity, finger strength, and motivation for hygiene may influence the prosthetic option. If the patient's dexterity for hygiene and his or her finances are not a consideration, the fixed mandibular implant prosthesis may be the treatment of choice.

With a prosthesis of any kind, advantages and disadvantages exist. The advantages of the mandibular fixed prosthesis compared with an implant-retained overdenture are as follows:

1. *Lack of tissue contact.* No mucosal support is required with the fixed prosthesis. The implant abutment unit supports the prosthesis completely, allowing no prosthetic movement. This eliminates any potential tissue irritation from prosthesis movement.
2. *Increased masticatory efficiency.* The implant-retained fixed prosthesis functions similarly to that of natural dentition. The only limitation to chewing is from the maxilla, if removable prosthetics are present.
3. *Psychologic advantage.* Tooth loss and the wearing of a complete denture are often associated with aging. Some patients have moderate-to-severe psychologic problems regarding edentulism or using a removable prosthesis. The fixed prosthesis eliminates a removable prosthesis and greatly enhances the patient's self-image and self-confidence.

Disadvantages of the fixed implant-supported prosthesis include the following:

1. *Lack of tissue support.* Many patients who have complete dentures have undergone considerable resorption of the mandible. The denture was used to reestablish lip support and facial contours. The mental labial fold has often been eliminated by the removable prosthesis, and the patient has become accustomed to this appearance. The tissue support provided by the fixed prosthesis may not provide the expected facial support. The length of the cantilever distance is measured from the distal surface of the distal-most fixture on each side. The maximum recommended cantilever is 15 mm. This distance may leave the patient in first molar occlusion and with a lack of tissue support in the mandibular posterior.
2. *Complicated procedures.* The clinical and laboratory procedures are technically more demanding with the fixed prosthesis compared with the overdenture prosthesis.
3. *Expense.* Surgical and prosthetic procedures may cost the patient several thousand dollars more than an overdenture or removable prosthesis for the following reasons:
   a. More implants and components are used.
   b. The number and length of clinical appointments for prosthetic completion are increased.
   c. The technical procedures in the laboratory are more

specialized, and a higher degree of expertise is required.

5. *Hygiene.* The contours of the implant prosthesis may prove difficult for patients with poor eyesight, limited dexterity, or lack of motivation to maintain a plaque-free environment.

CLINICAL AND LABORATORY PROCEDURES

Procedures for the mandibular fixed prosthesis begin 7 to 10 days after the fixture placements. The patient may need transitional denture fabricated before surgery to establish phonetics and esthetics at the proper vertical dimension of occlusion. The transitional denture is used to evaluate the patient's temporomandibular joint response to the vertical dimension of occlusion and as a guide for fabrication of the surgical stent. If the existing dentures are adequate, a transitional denture is not necessary. After sutures are removed and adequate tissue healing has occurred, a tissue conditioner is used to reline the mandibular denture. The denture is relieved in the area corresponding to the flap reflection. The tissue conditioning material is mixed and applied, the denture is seated, the border is molded, and the patient is guided into centric relation occlusion. After the recommended set time, the denture is removed and placed in a pressure pot at 20 pounds per square inch (psi) in warm water for 10 minutes. The excess material is trimmed, and the denture is polished. The denture is worn, and tissue-treatment material is replaced as needed until healing is complete. A processed methylmethacrylate resin reline is completed, and the denture is worn until the abutment surgery is performed. The patient is advised to seek denture adjustment for all tissue irritation to prevent implant exposure. For the mandible, 4 months is the average healing period before the abutment surgery is completed.

About 7 to 10 days after the abutment surgery, the mandibular denture is again tissue treated as previously described, except that now the denture is relieved adequately to allow for clearance around the abutments and the healing caps. Preliminary impressions of the maxilla and the mandible are made using an alginate impression material in stock edentulous impression trays (Figs. 3-1 and 3-2).

The preliminary alginate impression is poured in dental stone and trimmed for the preparation of the custom tray fabrication (Fig. 3-3).

Custom Tray Fabrication

The custom tray is used to make an impression that will provide an accurate recording of the mandibular or maxillary tissues and their relationship to the abutments. This tray is different from a standard edentulous tray in that it has openings that are designed to allow access to the guide pins and impression copings. The impression copings and guide pins are picked up in the impression material confined within the tray. This provides an accurate relationship of the abutments to one another and to surrounding oral tissues.

Baseplate wax is used to provide relief in the buccal, lingual, and distal areas to the abutments on the cast for custom tray fabrication (Fig. 3-4). A single layer of baseplate wax is used as a relief in the distal extension areas. Sufficient wax relief is achieved by a strip of baseplate wax 8 mm wide by 6 mm high (Fig. 3-5) over the crest of the residual ridge and over the abutment fixture area. The ridge is then smoothed with a wax spatula.

The custom tray material is molded over the cast, and the abutment area is reinforced with excess resin (Figs. 3-6 and 3-7). A laboratory knife is used to cut a window over the occlusal portion of the abutment relief area, which is then allowed to completely polymerize (Fig. 3-8).

After polymerization the custom tray is removed from the preliminary cast and the borders are trimmed similar to a conventional denture. The distal and lingual extension of the custom tray is cut short of the full denture border (Fig. 3-9). The tray is placed on the cast and verified for a minimum clearance of 3 mm between the custom tray and the replica area of the abutment. If the clearance is acceptable, it is polished and ready for final impressions (Fig. 3-10).

Final Impression Procedures

Titanium hemostats and the hexagonal wrench are used to ensure abutment screw tightness (Fig. 3-11). If abutment screws have loosened, one of the torque drivers is used to tighten all abutment screws. Impression copings are attached

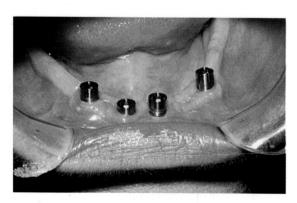

Figure 3-1

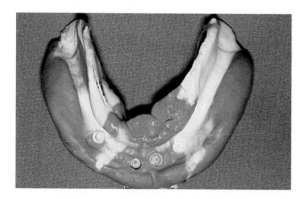

Figure 3-2

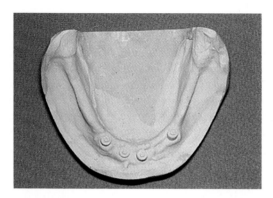

Figure 3-3

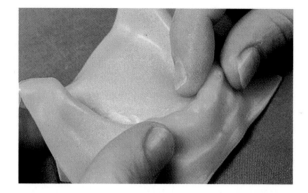

Figure 3-4

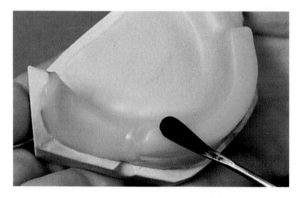

Figure 3-5

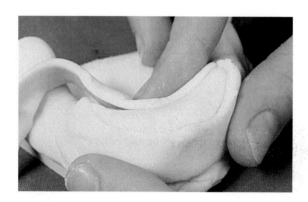

Figure 3-6

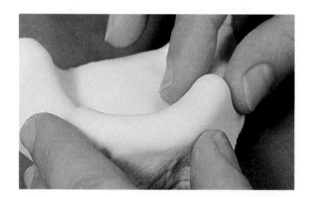

Figure 3-7

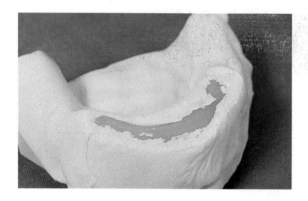

Figure 3-8

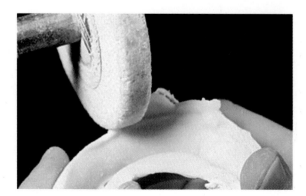

Figure 3-9

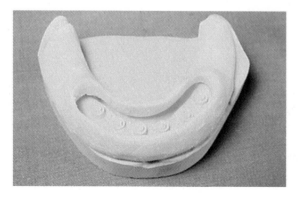

Figure 3-10

to the abutments with the proper length guide pins (Fig. 3-12). The square impression copings are preferred because they resist rotation and displacement in the impression material. The open window custom tray is tried in the mouth for comfort and path of insertion (Fig. 3-13). The abutment, impression coping, and guide pin angulation and/or interference may necessitate adjustment of the tray dimension to allow insertion. Baseplate wax is sealed over the window, and the tray is heated in a water bath and then inserted over the guide pins and impression copings (Fig. 3-14).

The guide pins should penetrate the wax to allow access for removal of the impression (Figs. 3-15 and 3-16). The tray

is painted with the appropriate adhesive, and the impression material of choice is mixed to manufacturer's specifications. The impression material should be a medium viscosity mix that will flow through a syringe and should have a stiff set (Fig. 3-17). A vinyl polysiloxane impression material is recommended. After the impression is mixed, the material is loaded into the tray and the syringe. The material is first injected around the impression copings, and the tray is seated, using the guide pins and holes in the wax window as a guide for placement. Ideally, the guide pins should all penetrate the wax window, and the screw slots in the guide pins should be accessible. Excess impression material is cleared from the

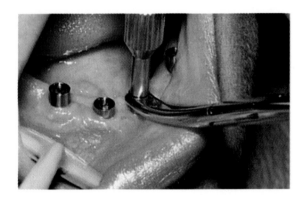

Figure 3-11

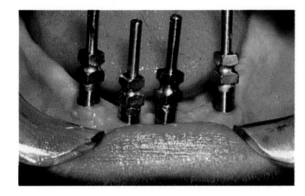

Figure 3-12

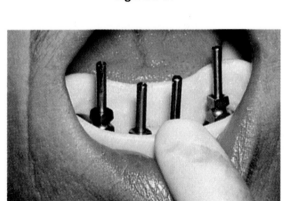

Figure 3-13

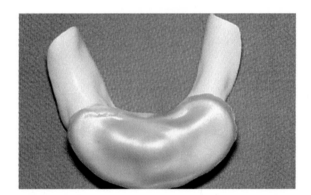

Figure 3-14

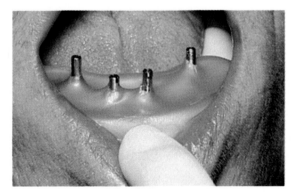

Figure 3-15

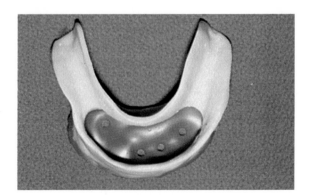

Figure 3-16

guide pins before complete setting. After the impression material has set, the guide pins are accessed and then unscrewed with a screwdriver of the appropriate length (Figs. 3-18 and 3-19). The guide pins are unscrewed until two or three clicks are heard, which indicates a complete guide pin disconnection. The guide pins are left in the same holes in the impression to allow for accurate placement of the abutment replicas. Final impressions of the maxilla are also completed at this time.

Master Cast

The master cast is the foundation for fabricating the implant prosthesis. Therefore the dental technician must use methodic procedures that will ensure an accurate reproduction of the intraoral tissues.

Brass replicas have been precisely machined to be analogs of the superior surface of the abutment. The replicas are screwed onto the impression copings with guide pins. Extreme caution must be used not to entrap any foreign material between the brass replica and the impression coping interface. Foreign material may cause inaccuracy in the master cast, which is subsequently transferred to the framework.

After the placement of the brass replicas, the final impression is beaded with utility wax and boxed with wax strips in the usual manner (Fig. 3-20). The impression is cast in vacuum-mixed diestone. Retention for the second pour is then placed in the distal extension areas (Fig. 3-21). The anterior region around the replicas is left flat for cast alterations (if necessary) after the framework trial fitting. When the first pour has set, a base in yellow stone is poured (Fig. 3-22). Each guide pin must then be completely unscrewed until the characteristic click is heard two or three times before separating the impression from the cast. Elimination of this step may result in fracturing to the cast or damage to the impression.

Occlusion Rim Fabrication

Maxillomandibular relationships are recorded using a customized record base and an interocclusal rim. The record base is stabilized by incorporating gold cylinders or impression copings into the record base. This base is unique because it can be secured in the mouth with guide pins for recording centric relation and vertical dimension of occlusion.

The occlusion rim is fabricated on the master cast. Gold cylinders or impression copings are placed on two or three of the abutment replicas on the master cast. Placement on the anterior abutments facilitates access during clinical trial fittings.

One thickness of baseplate wax is adapted around the replicas and extended slightly beyond the most distal replicas. Three replicas are located and exposed through the block-

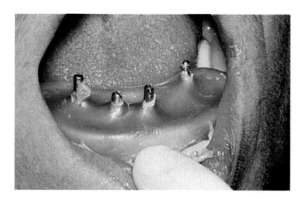

Figure 3-17

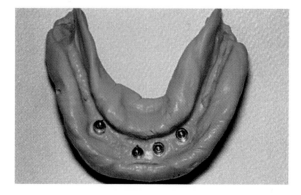

Figure 3-18

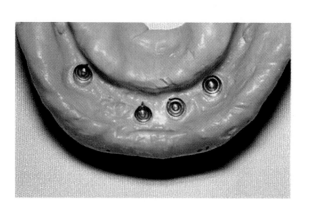

Figure 3-19

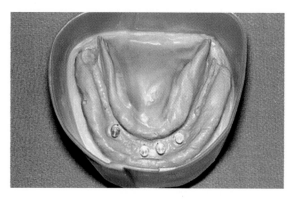

Figure 3-20

out wax, and guide pins are screwed into the impression copings (Figs. 3-23 and 3-24).

Undesirable undercuts on the master cast are blocked out with baseplate wax. A tinfoil substitute is placed on the exposed areas of the stone, and an autopolymerizing resin is mixed according to manufacturer's directions, rolled out, and adapted to the master cast (Fig. 3-25). The tray material must engage undercuts in the gold cylinders or impression copings. A double thickness of resin is added to the lingual area of the occlusion rim. The additional bulk of material is important for strength on the distal extension areas. A laboratory scalpel is used to clear the facial areas of the acrylic

resin around the brass replicas and impression copings, exposing their interface. This interface is used to verify complete seating of the occlusion rim during maxillomandibular relations. When the acrylic resin record base has completely polymerized, it is carefully separated from the cast, and the relief wax is removed with a laboratory knife. The interface between the brass replica and the gold cylinder is opened for visualization on the facial surfaces. The borders of the record base are trimmed and polished (Fig. 3-26). The record base is placed on the working cast, guide pins are reinserted, and accuracy of the abutment coping interface is verified (Fig. 3-27). Baseplate wax is used to fabricate the occlusion rim in

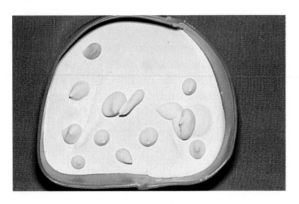

Figure 3-21

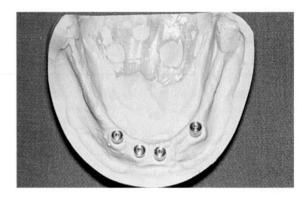

Figure 3-22

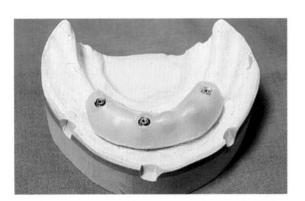

Figure 3-23

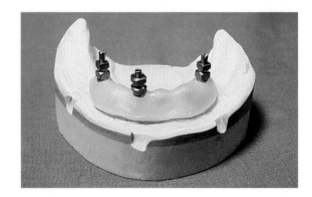

Figure 3-24

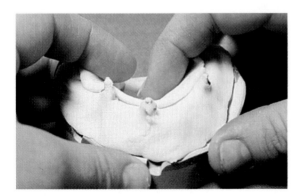

Figure 3-25

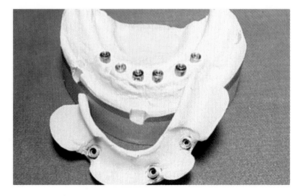

Figure 3-26

the usual fashion (Fig. 3-28). The mandibular occlusion rim can be fabricated initially to average dimensions (18 mm high anteriorly by 8 mm wide posteriorly). Access to each of the guide pins is created through the surface of the wax rim. The guide pins can be modified, either at this stage or by the restorative dentist, when the maxillomandibular relations are recorded. This is done so that the guide pins do not interfere with recording the correct occlusal vertical dimension and centric relation. The edges of the wax are finished to create smooth surfaces, and the accuracy of the interface between the coping and replica is rechecked (Fig. 3-29).

Maxillomandibular Relations

Wax occlusion rims are used to establish maxillomandibular relations in the usual fashion. The mandibular occlusion rim is stabilized with gold copings or altered impression copings (Fig. 3-30). Centric relation records, protrusive records, and a facebow registration are made (Fig. 3-31). At this appointment, tooth shade and denture tooth mold are selected, and the occlusal scheme is selected, depending on the nature of the maxillary arch and its relationship with the mandible.

Esthetic Trial Fitting

The casts are mounted on a semiadjustable articulator using the facebow and centric relation records. The protrusive record is used for setting the condylar inclination. The wax

occlusion rims are used as a guide for setting the denture teeth. Anterior (Figs. 3-32 and 3-33) and full-tooth trial fittings are used to establish esthetics, phonetics, lip support, and the proper vertical dimension of occlusion. Centric relation is also verified with the interocclusal records.

The maximum distal extension cantilever is 15 mm distal to the distal-most fixture abutment unit bilaterally. The distance is modified by the following factors:

1. *Arch form of abutment.* Implant placement in a straight line places more load on the implants, abutments, abutment screws, and all components than does placement with an arch form. The cantilever is shortened to 10 mm.
2. *Implant length and prognosis.* Distal implants shorter than 10 mm (or those placed in less-than-ideal bone) limit load potential, and cantilever extension is shortened to 10 mm.
3. *Anterior cantilever.* Class II jaw relationships and lingual fixture placement may necessitate an anterior cantilever for proper tooth arrangement. Three separate cantilevered sections may be necessary (two distal, one anterior) for proper tooth arrangement. This increases the load on all implants and prosthetic components. The distal cantilever should be shortened in this situation.
4. *Natural maxillary dentition.* Natural maxillary dentition opposing the implant prosthesis applies more load to the

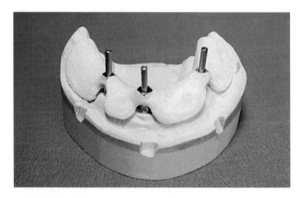

Figure 3-27

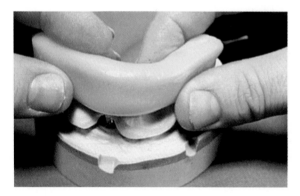

Figure 3-28

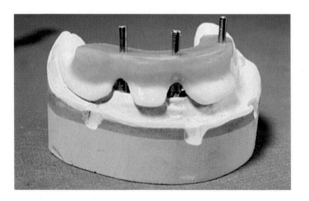

Figure 3-29

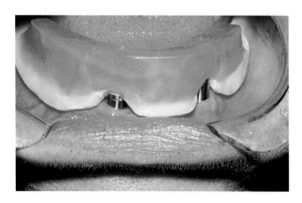

Figure 3-30

mandibular prosthesis, and cantilevers should be shortened to 10 mm.

5. *Parafunctional habits.* Clenching and bruxism add an additional load to implants and prosthetic components. Shortening distal cantilevers and fabrication of a nightguard will lessen the load on components. Before the framework is designed, the surgeon and the restorative dentist should discuss and record the implant length and the quality of bone found at the implant placement. Other parameters are evaluated, and the final cantilever distances are used during tooth trial fittings and discussed with the dental technician for framework design. Excess cantilevers overload the implants and components. Possible consequences of overload include fixture loss and component loosening and fracture. (See complications in Chapter 14.)

A survey of the master cast establishes the parameters used to determine both the symmetry and maximal extension of the distal portion of the implant-retained prosthesis (Figs. 3-34 and 3-35).

After completion of preliminary denture setup, it is necessary to drill a vertical hole through selective denture teeth to gain access to the underlying fixture. The baseplate wax is removed from beneath the denture tooth, and the alignment of the implant is determined using the guide pin. A #10 round

bur mounted in a straight handpiece is used to create a vertical access opening in the denture tooth, or the wax baseplate, to expose the brass replica (Fig. 3-36 and 3-37).

The completed prosthetic setup is evaluated in the usual fashion (Fig. 3-38). All maxillomandibular relations are reverified, and the occlusal contacts are reconfirmed at this session (Fig. 3-39). The setup is returned to the dental laboratory where the construction of the framework will begin.

The patient is invited to have a friend or significant other help in esthetic evaluation. The mandibular setup can be secured to two abutments for stability during evaluation. The patient must be totally happy with cosmetics and final facial support before framework fabrication.

FRAMEWORK FABRICATION
Matrix Fabrication

A vinyl polysiloxane elastomer putty or laboratory plaster matrix is fabricated on the trial tooth setup to preserve the relationship of the teeth and waxing to the underlying cast framework.

The superior portion of the cast base is indexed in the following three areas: the anterior midline, the right posterior molar region, and the left posterior molar region (Fig. 3-40). A grinding wheel mounted on a low-speed dental handpiece is used to complete this procedure. Indexing the cast in three diverse areas ensures that the matrix can be

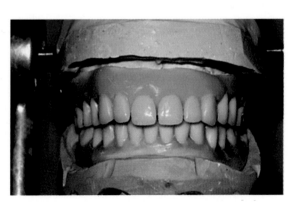

Figure 3-31

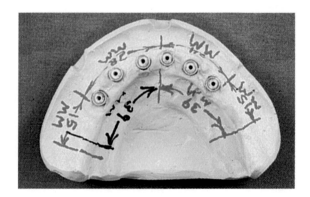

Figure 3-32

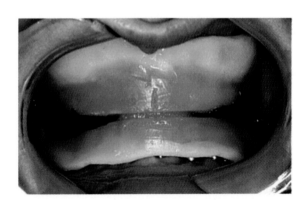

Figure 3-33

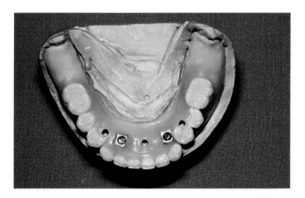

Figure 3-34

replaced on the cast in a firm, predictable position. The interproximal areas between the denture teeth are opened using a wax carving instrument (Fig. 3-41). This allows the matrix material to flow readily between the teeth. It also makes it easier to position and hold the denture teeth in the matrix for repositioning on the framework. The medium-viscosity putty is mixed according to the manufacturer's directions and in sufficient quantity to be placed around the buccal and the labial aspects and over the occlusal aspect of the denture setup. When the material is ready, it is molded across the anterior labial and the posterior buccal surfaces of the setup,

forcing the material between the interproximal areas and into the indexing grooves on the cast base (Fig. 3-42). The material is worked across the teeth and around the guide pins. The completed matrix has impression material molded on all sides of the denture wax-up and the guide pins; only the tips of the guide pins are left exposed (Fig. 3-43). This procedure creates a positive orientation between the cast and the wax-up.

A sectional plaster matrix is an alternative technique. The matrix is removed from the master cast, and the excess impression material is trimmed from the lingual surface of

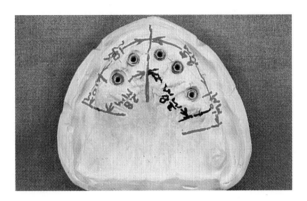

Figure 3-35

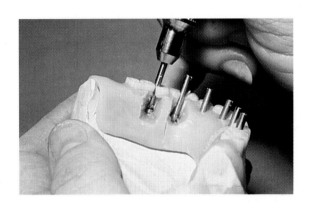

Figure 3-36

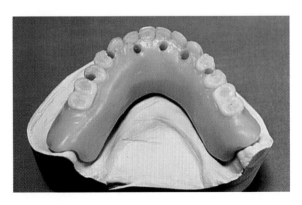

Figure 3-37

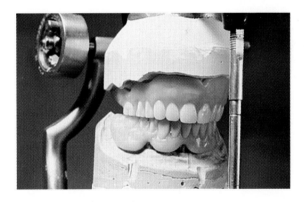

Figure 3-38

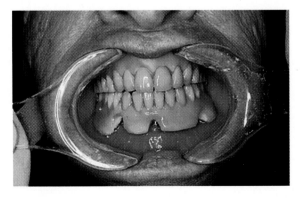

Figure 3-39

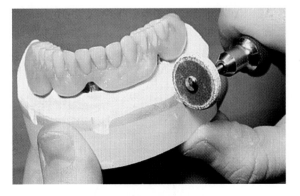

Figure 3-40

the wax-up using a laboratory scalpel (Fig. 3-44). This area is removed from both the anterior and posterior lingual surfaces to give full access to the lingual surfaces during subsequent waxing procedures. The notched areas provide the positive orientation of the cast on the labial aspect of the impression material. The denture teeth are carefully removed from the tooth arrangement (Fig. 3-45). Any wax residue is removed with boiling water and then flushed with a mild detergent. The teeth are rinsed and dried before replacing them into the matrix. All of the individual denture teeth are replaced into the matrix and held in place with a dab of sticky wax that is placed on a cusp tip or an incisal edge. The wax

must be kept away from the guide pin holes. The matrix is placed back onto the master cast when the teeth have been secured (Fig. 3-46). Adequate clearance between the guide pins and the denture teeth is verified.

FRAMEWORK WAX-UP

The implant components used in the framework waxing procedure are the guide pin, gold cylinder and screw, and the brass replica/analog (Fig. 3-47). To stabilize the gold cylinders and minimize warpage of the wax pattern, a verification splint may be fabricated. When using the fine-grained resin, make cuts between several sections, replace them on the cast, and

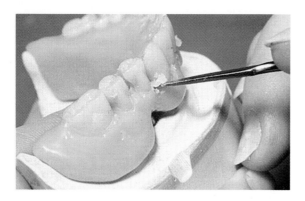

Figure 3-41

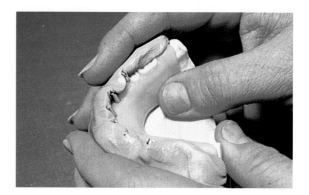

Figure 3-42

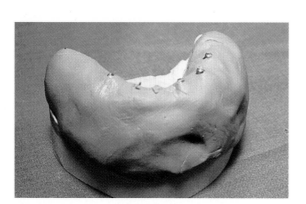

Figure 3-43

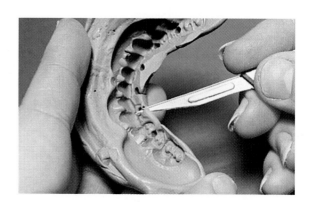

Figure 3-44

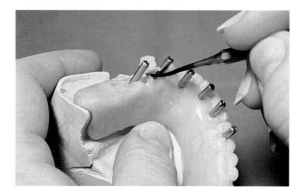

Figure 3-45

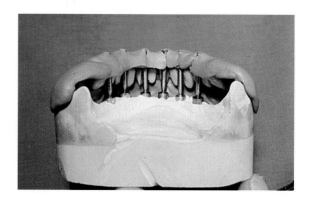

Figure 3-46

secure them with new material to minimize internal stress. The substructure waxing is replaced on the master cast and secured with guide pins. The area below and around the abutment analogs is blocked out with modeling compound. Modeling compound is extended distally to the predetermined maximum extensions of the prosthetic framework. A small trough is created at the distal extension areas to be used as a receptacle for wax; the trough will control the flow of the wax and minimize the amount of wax used (Fig. 3-48). A wax-separating medium is applied to the denture teeth within the matrix; this facilitates removal of the teeth from the framework waxing. The wax portion of the framework is fabricated quickly by luring the matrix to the cast with sticky wax or cyanoacrylate adhesive (Fig. 3-49). The gold cylinders, matrix, and splint are stabilized with the long lubricated guide pins. A glass eyedropper is filled with molten wax; the molten wax flows into the matrix over the luted denture teeth and the gold cylinders and then flows into the trough (Fig. 3-50). The wax is allowed to solidify at room temperature without applying any external coolant (Fig. 3-51). The waxing *must not* be chilled with cold water or cooled with compressed air because this may cause an internal stress formation within the wax pattern. The matrix is removed, and any modeling compound is cleaned from the master cast and waxing (Fig. 3-52). The waxing is replaced on the master

cast, and a reference line is placed on the side of the master cast base for each denture tooth midline. The line will serve as a guide for placement of retentive struts that will not interfere with the resetting of the denture teeth (Fig. 3-53).

Excess wax is cleared from around the gold cylinders and the distal extension areas of the waxing (Figs. 3-54 and 3-55). The labial and lingual interproximal areas are opened around each of the abutment replicas, and convex contours are carved around the gold cylinders to allow sufficient space for hygiene (Fig. 3-56). The lingual contour is carved to allow room for the tongue. Excessive contour may interfere with speech. *Caution:* when completing the wax-up, try to work with the pattern on the master cast as much as possible. Handling of the fragile wax pattern might cause distortion or breakage.

The cantilevered pontic area of the waxing is positioned directly distal to the last abutment and is connected to the last cylinder with a J-shaped connector. The shape of this portion of the wax-up is important because it contributes to the strength of the distal extension. *Excessive cutback beyond the J-section may lead to fracture of the framework.* The ideal dimension of this J-section is 4 mm wide by 6 mm high (24 mm^2). The pontic, connected to the J-section (Fig. 3-57), is positioned 1 to 2 mm above the tissues of the posterior residual ridge to prevent tissue hyperplasia and to allow room for adequate hygiene procedures (Fig. 3-58). The wax is

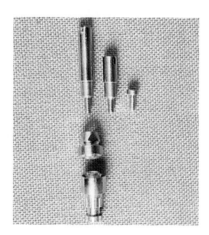

Figure 3-47

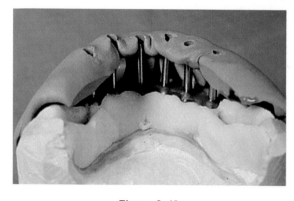

Figure 3-48

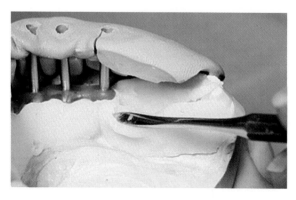

Figure 3-49

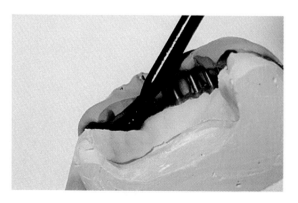

Figure 3-50

smoothed and sealed around the gold cylinders. This is achieved by lightly polishing the waxing with a cotton-tipped applicator moistened with Xylene (Fig. 3-59). Any wax residue from the inferior surface of the gold cylinders must be removed; otherwise there may be casting flash over these areas. Xylene is used sparingly because it is a powerful solvent. It is used because it produces an even, smooth texture to the wax pattern (Fig. 3-60). After the complete waxing has been smoothed, the lingual surface of each distal extension section is marked for a wax cutback. A metal/acrylic resin finishing line is created halfway between the occlusal surface and the inferior border of the distal cantilevered sec-

tion. The prosthesis waxing should be cut back one half of that distance. There are many different configurations to the lingual surface of the implant prosthesis wax-up, but the overriding consideration should be one of maintaining the strength of the casting. In the anterior lingual region, the metal/acrylic resin finishing line is designed anterior to the placement of the guide pins; this facilitates the procedure because it allows screw access in metal when removing the prosthesis at a later date (Fig. 3-61). On the labial and buccal surfaces a 1 to 2 mm finishing line is carved above the gold cylinders (Fig. 3-62). The wax pattern is hollowed out with a bur to provide maximum room for retention of the acrylic

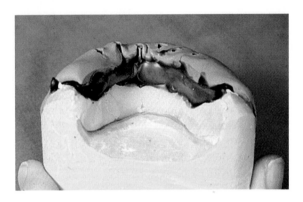

Figure 3-51

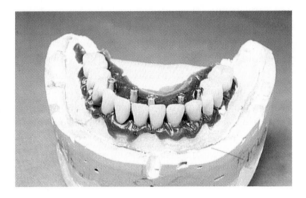

Figure 3-52

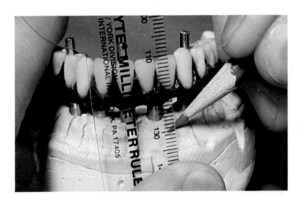

Figure 3-53

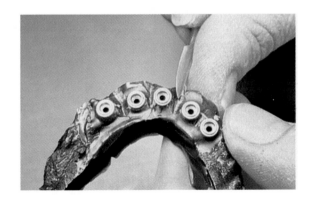

Figure 3-54

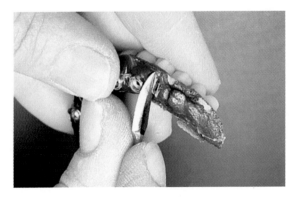

Figure 3-55

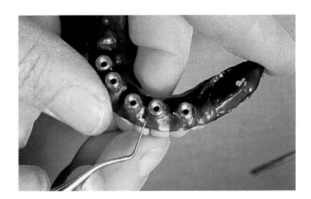

Figure 3-56

resin (Fig. 3-63). The interproximal areas are scalloped to allow a minimal amount of metal to be visible on the labial surface. In the distal extension areas, a minimum 24 mm² of metal must be maintained. There are four methods of providing retention to the cutback wax pattern: (1) undercuts placed around the guide pins, (2) 18-gauge wax retention bar placement, (3) application of plastic retention beads, and (4) bonding agents. With the wax pattern placed on the master cast, the predetermined reference marks are used to place 18-gauge wax strips in a vertical correspondence to the midline of the denture teeth (Fig. 3-64). Plastic retentive beads are also placed on the internal surfaces of the wax pat-

tern for additional retention. A tacky liquid should be used on the portions of the wax-up to receive plastic beads (Fig. 3-65) before they are applied.

SPRUING

An indirect feeder bar spruing method is used in the casting of the prosthesis framework. A 6-gauge plastic feeder bar is heated, allowed to soften, and then bent to the arch form of the waxing (Fig. 3-66). The posterior ends are cross-stabilized with another piece of 6-gauge plastic feeder bar (Fig. 3-67). Eight-gauge wax sprues that are 3 to 4 mm long are secured to the waxing between the guide pin holes, and two sprues are

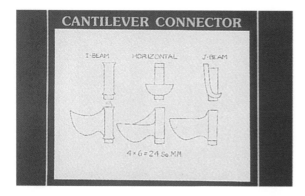

Figure 3-57

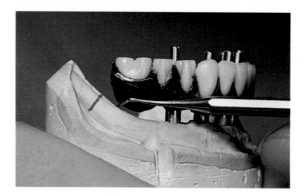

Figure 3-58

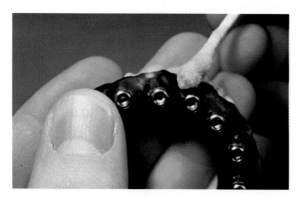

Figure 3-59

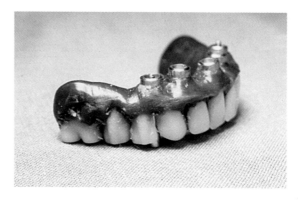

Figure 3-60

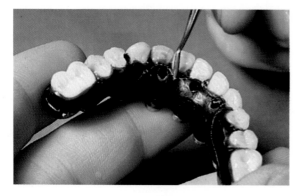

Figure 3-61

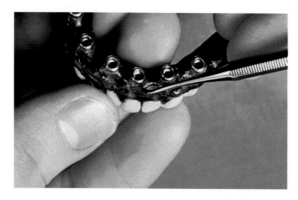

Figure 3-62

placed on each distal extension. A 6-gauge sprue is attached to the distal extension for cross-arch stabilization (Fig. 3-68). The size of the plastic feeder bar is determined by the bulky part of the waxing. The stabilized bar is coated with wax before it is attached to the sprues. Coating the bar with wax allows the wax to be eliminated through the sprue holes before the plastic bar is burned out and eliminates the entrapment of wax in the investment. Four 6-gauge auxiliary sprues are then placed and angled indirectly for the attachment of the wax pattern to the sprue-former base (Fig. 3-69). The indirect spruing technique will ensure an even flow of molten alloy into the mold cavity. The completed sprued wax pattern

is weighed to determine the amount of alloy necessary to complete the casting (Fig. 3-70). The wax pattern is placed on the sprue former, and a distal extension reference point is marked (Figs. 3-71 and 3-72). The gold cylinders are cleaned with an ammonia solution to remove any residual oil or other residue that might cause casting flash (Fig. 3-73). A casting ring that weighs 400 to 600 grams is lined with a nonasbestos liner.

SELECTING THE CASTING ALLOY

A variety of metals may be used to cast the framework: ceramic, gold, or palladium-silver alloys. However, the metal

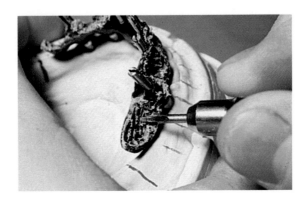

Figure 3-63

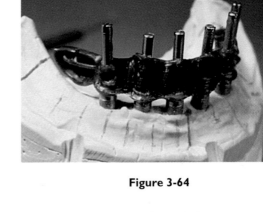

Figure 3-64

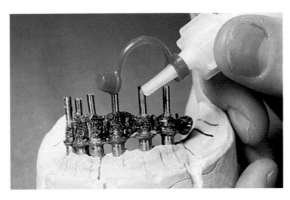

Figure 3-65

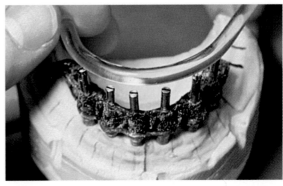

Figure 3-66

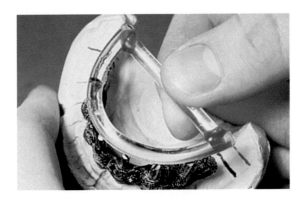

Figure 3-67

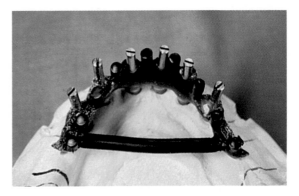

Figure 3-68

that is selected must meet a minimum tensile strength of 60,000 psi. In the United States the use of a palladium-silver alloy is preferred, primarily because of cost factors. The chosen alloy should be able to be cast at a temperature below 2300° F. The gold cylinders will be damaged if the casting temperature is higher than 2300° F. The method used to determine the amount of alloy needed to ensure a complete casting is determined by the following formula:

$$\text{Wax weight} \times \text{Specific gravity} = \text{Amount of alloy needed}$$
$$(\text{e.g., } 3.75 \text{ DWT} \times 10.6 = 39.75 \text{ DWT})$$

The amount of metal required is governed by the specific gravity of the alloy, and this is determined by the manufacturer. Using this formula reduces the costly error associated with using either too little or too much alloy for the casting.

INVESTING THE WAX PATTERN

Orient the waxing in the selected casting ring, leaving 10 to 13 mm of space all around the pattern for investment. Allow for at least 6 mm of investment over the top of the waxing (Fig. 3-74). The sprue-former base is marked to orient the distal extension portion of the pattern so that it can be correctly aligned in the cradle of the casting machine. When the ring is cast, it should be arranged in the centrifugal casting machine with the marked distal extensions in a trailing posi-

tion. A high-heat, phosphate-bound investment is used with a powder/liquid ratio to achieve maximum expansion when palladium-silver alloy or other similar metal is cast. The investment is poured into the casting ring statically; the clinician must be careful not to entrap air in the guide pin holes because the investment must come up through the holes (Fig. 3-75).

CASTING THE WAX PATTERN

A two-stage burnout system is recommended when using the large investment rings. When oxygen and natural gas are used, the oxygen pressure is set at 15 to 20 pounds, and the ring is cast after burnout in a normal fashion. Make sure that the distal extension portion of the casting ring is placed in the trailing position of the machine's cradle.

FINISHING THE CASTING

The casting is roughly broken out from the investment, and the clinician must be careful to protect the gold cylinders and the inferior surface of the casting. *Do not use any abrasives that will cause damage to the inferior surfaces or the gold cylinders.* The casting is cleaned with aluminum oxide or glass beads, protecting the gold cylinders (Figs. 3-76 and 3-77). Protection caps placed over the cylinders help eliminate possible damage. The framework is removed from the feeder sprues and stabilizing bar using a separating disc

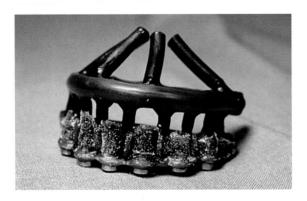

Figure 3-69

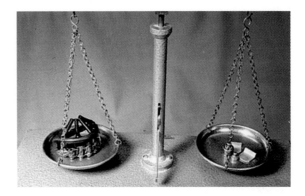

Figure 3-70

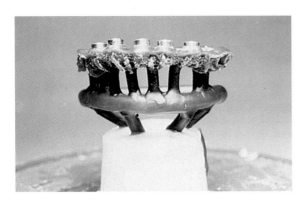

Figure 3-71

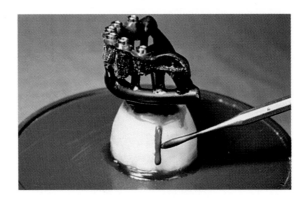

Figure 3-72

mounted on a low-speed handpiece (Fig. 3-78). A #10 round bur is used to remove investment from the guide pin holes, being careful not to damage the seat of the gold cylinders (Figs. 3-79 and 3-80). Damage to the gold cylinder seat will keep the prosthesis from seating accurately. After each guide pin hole has been cleaned, the casting is placed on the master cast and checked circumferentially for interface accuracy between each brass replica and gold cylinder. Complete interface accuracy should be established with one guide pin screwed in place anywhere on the casting (Figs. 3-81 and 3-82). The casting can then be returned to the clinic for a trial fitting.

FRAMEWORK TRIAL FITTING

The abutments are thoroughly cleaned, and the titanium hemostats and hexagonal wrench are used to confirm abutment tightness. The framework is tried on the abutments using only passive tightening of the gold alloy screws in an incremental tightening pattern (Fig. 3-83). The abutment framework-interface should show intimate and circumferential contact for all abutments. Tenderness during tightening may indicate improper fit. If pain is elicited at this time, it may indicate an ill-fitting framework. If the patient reports sensitivity in one of the distal fixtures, this may also indicate proximity to the mental nerve. A mirror must be used to

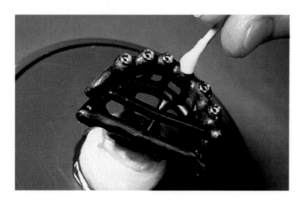

Figure 3-73

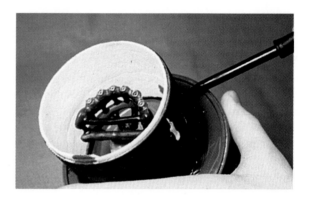

Figure 3-74

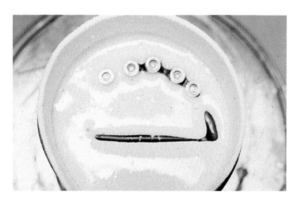

Figure 3-75

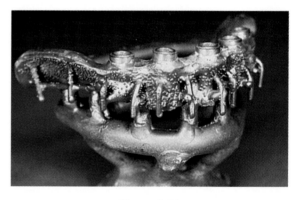

Figure 3-76

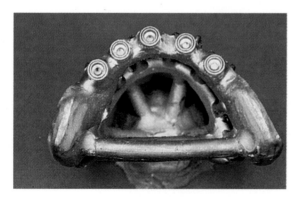

Figure 3-77

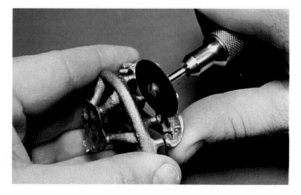

Figure 3-78

check for intimate fit. If the interface inaccuracy is noticed, the framework must be sectioned around the ill-fitting segment. The framework is removed from the mouth and sectioned using an ultrafine separating disc. Care should be taken to keep the cut no greater than 0.4 mm for ease of soldering. The sectioned framework is tried in the mouth to ensure intimate fit between all abutments and the framework. The segments are aligned, making sure that there is no metal contact between sections (Fig. 3-84).

The sections are lured with autopolymerizing resin while secured in the mouth (Fig. 3-85). This can be accomplished by filling a syringe with mixed resin and inserting the resin

into each of the sectioned areas. A straight handpiece bur can be used to cross-arch stabilize the framework in the mouth. The resined framework is allowed to polymerize, the guide pins are removed, and the sectioned, resin-secured framework is returned to the laboratory for soldering.

SOLDERING

If the casting does not accurately fit the master cast as previously described or if it does not seat completely upon clinical trial fitting, the casting must be sectioned and the framework parts must be soldered together in the laboratory. Since the casting no longer fits the master cast, the cast is altered to

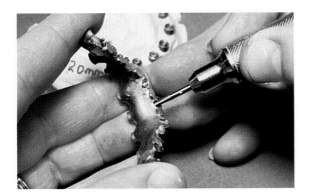

Figure 3-79

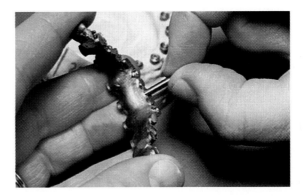

Figure 3-80

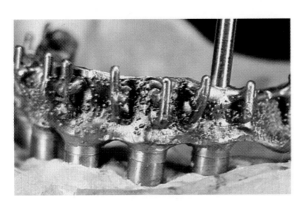

Figure 3-81

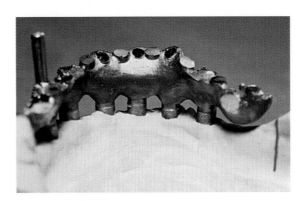

Figure 3-82

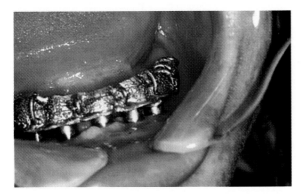

Figure 3-83

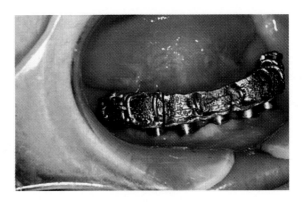

Figure 3-84

fit the casting (Fig. 3-86). The brass replicas corresponding to the altered section of the framework are removed from the master cast with a separating disc (Figs. 3-87 to 3-89). Residual stone is removed from around each misaligned replica and replaced on the framework; the framework is then remounted with the guide pin screws on the master cast. Complete relief around each replica is verified (Fig. 3-90). A small portion of diestone is mixed and placed around the brass replicas (Fig. 3-91) and allowed to set. The autopolymerizing resin is removed from the casting by heating it over an open Bunsen burner flame. Each of the cleaned segments is replaced on this adjusted master cast.

To stabilize the framework segments, sticky wax is flowed into each joint place to be soldered, and a bar is placed across the arch to reach each solder joint (Fig. 3-92). The sticky wax is chilled by running the cast under cold water. Additional sticky wax is placed on the inferior surfaces of the solder joint areas. *Extreme care is taken to not get sticky wax on the gold cylinder surface or interface, or solder will flash over these areas.* The framework is placed in soldering investment and allowed to set (Fig. 3-93). The sticky wax is removed by flushing the investment with boiling water; then the surfaces are cleaned with a detergent. The investment is relieved to provide access to the joints that are to be soldered (Fig. 3-94).

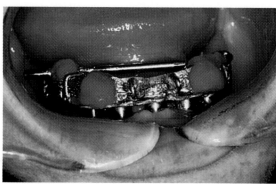

Figure 3-85

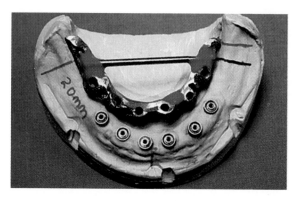

Figure 3-86

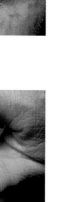

Figure 3-87

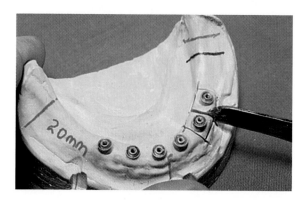

Figure 3-88

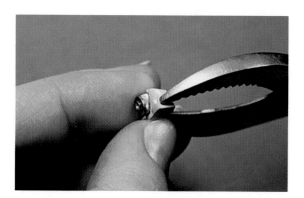

Figure 3-89

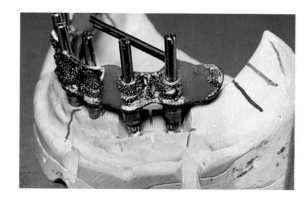

Figure 3-90

Soldering flux is placed in the joint space, and the investment is preheated for an even expansion. When each joint is soldered, the investment is heated from the labial aspect and solder is placed on the lingual surface and allowed to pull through from the lingual surface to the labial surface (Fig. 3-95). The soldered framework and investment are allowed to cool at room temperature. The casting is removed from the investment, cleaned, remounted on the altered master cast, and checked for the interface seating of the casting to the brass replicas.

POLISHING THE FRAMEWORK

Before any abrasive cleaning or finishing of the casting is done, the gold cylinders should be protected with protection caps or altered brass replicas (Fig. 3-96). *Negligence in this area may cause damage to the interface surfaces* (Fig. 3-97). *This is one of the most critical steps in the prosthesis fabrication. Failure to protect the interface surfaces at this point will result in destroying the seat of the prosthesis.* The retentive area of the brass replica is removed using a separating disc mounted in a low-speed handpiece (Fig. 3-98). This allows the dental technician to gain access to the undersurface and the interproximal areas of the framework to use a rubber wheel and polish the frame without damaging the gold cylinders. This protective measure should be used when cleaning with an air abrasive and finishing both the metal framework and the subsequent acrylic resin (Fig. 3-99). The final framework can be smoothed by using a number of different finishing methods and materials. Rubber wheels and/or points mounted in a low-speed handpiece are used to finish the framework (Fig. 3-100). The metal/acrylic resin finishing line is smoothed and finished using a carbide bur mounted in a high-speed handpiece (Fig. 3-101). The final high shine is imparted to the framework using a felt wheel and polishing compound. After the casting is finished and polished, it is ultrasonically cleaned and replaced on the working cast.

REEVALUATION OF FRAMEWORK FIT

The framework is again seated in the mouth passively, and the abutment framework interface is evaluated as described previously (Fig. 3-102). Visual inspection is used to verify intimate 360-degree contact between all abutment framework interfaces. The screws are tightened, and the patient is asked to report any pain as the framework is tightened. Either a mechanical or electric torque wrench is used to tighten to 10 Ncm. If the interfaces are accurate and no pain is elicited, the framework is removed in preparation for adding denture teeth. If the framework is ill fitting, it is again sectioned, indexed, and soldered until accurate fit is achieved. The fit of

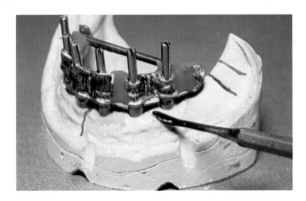

Figure 3-91

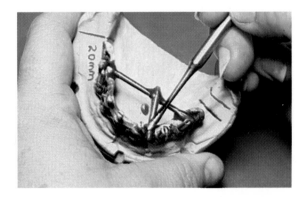

Figure 3-92

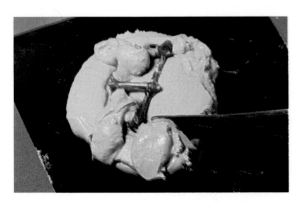

Figure 3-93

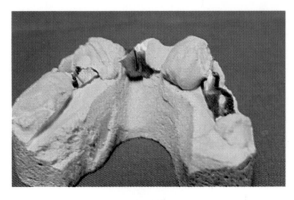

Figure 3-94

the framework is crucial to the long-term success of the prosthesis; many problems can be caused by an ill-fitting framework (see Chapter 14).

DENTURE TOOTH WAXING

The denture teeth are replaced into the vinyl polysiloxane matrix using sticky wax. The exact placement of the teeth is reconfirmed by comparing the tooth position with reference marks that have been placed on the side of the master cast.

Additional mechanical retention should be replaced in each denture tooth to ensure strong mechanical and chemical bonding of the denture tooth to the processed acrylic resin. Either a #2 or a #4 round bur mounted in a low-speed handpiece is used to drill small holes into the lingual surface of each denture tooth (Fig. 3-103). This is completed before the teeth are placed in the matrix. The matrix is replaced on the master cast containing the finished framework (Fig. 3-104). The denture teeth should not interfere with any of the retentive features (e.g., struts, beads). A glass eyedropper filled with molten baseplate wax is used to flow the molten wax between the teeth and casting incrementally until the matrix is filled. The wax is allowed to solidify (Fig. 3-105). The

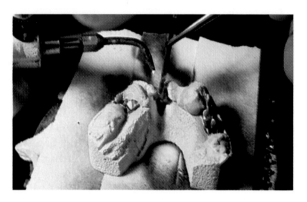

Figure 3-95

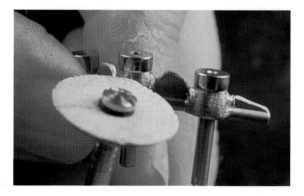

Figure 3-96

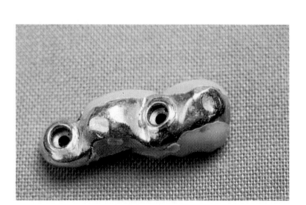

Figure 3-97

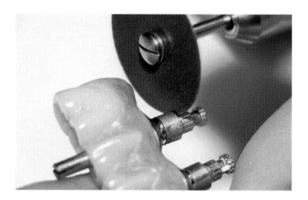

Figure 3-98

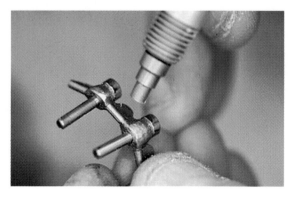

Figure 3-99

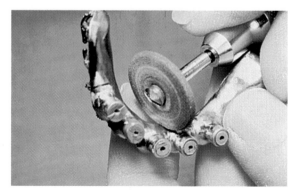

Figure 3-100

matrix is removed, and the areas around the denture teeth are carved and festooned. The occlusal contacts are checked and reestablished with the casts on the articulator.

FULL TRIAL TOOTH ARRANGEMENT ON FRAMEWORK

The full trial tooth arrangement on the maxillary occlusion rim and the mandibular framework is assessed in a final evaluation of all maxillomandibular relations. The patient is asked to closely evaluate the esthetics before the processing of the prostheses (Fig. 3-106). At this time it may be helpful to

have a family member or personal friend of the patient evaluate the esthetics also. After the patient approves the prosthesis, a centric relation record is made, and the prosthesis is ready for processing.

ACRYLIC PROCESSING AND FINAL FINISHING THE FRAMEWORK

Three methods are used in processing the denture teeth to the framework: (1) conventional trial packing and processing, (2) injection mold processing, and (3) light-cured composite processing. (Because of the complex steps that ensure total

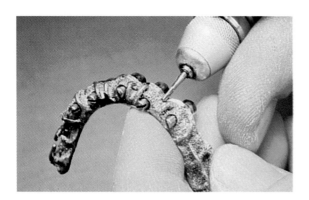

Figure 3-101

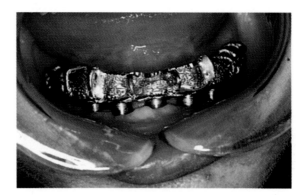

Figure 3-102

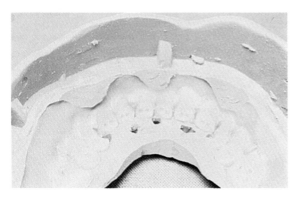

Figure 3-103

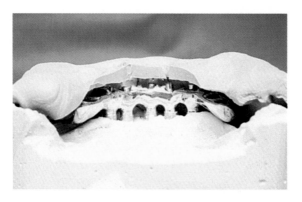

Figure 3-104

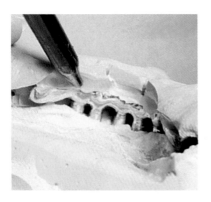

Figure 3-105

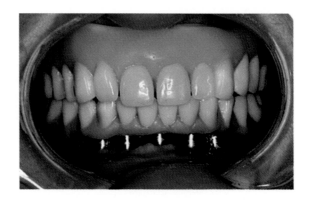

Figure 3-106

polymerization of the light-cured resin, along with the labor intensity to hand layer and manipulate the material before processing, light-cured composite processing is not a preferred method.) The conventional trial packing method is adequate, but problems may arise if the guide pins are not parallel; as a result, trial packing may have to be eliminated (Figs. 3-107 to 3-109). The injection mold processing, such as Ivoclar (Ivocap system), is the most desirable. Because the denture material is injected and cured under high pressure,

the methylmethacrylate resin is denser. Changes in occlusion after processing are minimal.

The prosthesis and master cast are invested in the bottom half of a denture flask (Fig. 3-110), and then the rest of the flasking procedure is completed in a normal method. The flask is placed in a boilout tank, is heated, and the wax is removed (Fig. 3-111). Both halves of the denture flask, mold cavity, and denture teeth are scrubbed, cleaned, and allowed to cool. A bonding agent may be applied to the frame to

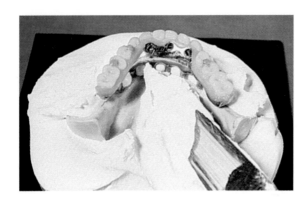

Figure 3-107

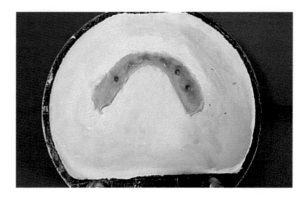

Figure 3-108

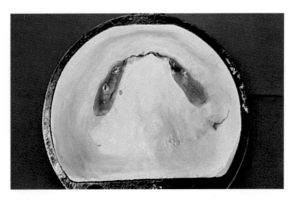

Figure 3-109

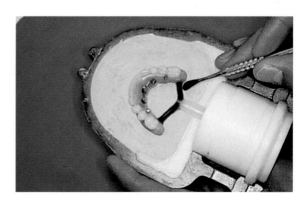

Figure 3-110

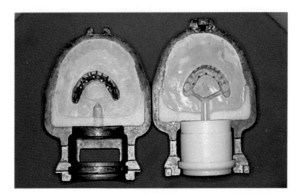

Figure 3-111

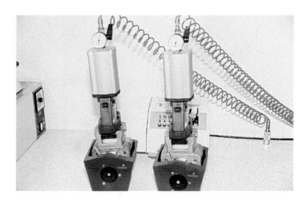

Figure 3-112

enhance the bond between the methylmethacrylate resin and the metal. The bonding agent *must not* be applied to the exposed area of the guide pins, or the guide pins will become permanently bonded. It is also recommended to apply a tissue-tinted opaque to mask out the darkness of the cast frame, which will enhance gingival tone.

The prosthesis is processed using a standard curing cycle recommended by the manufacturer (Fig. 3-112). The prosthesis is carefully removed from the flask. A laboratory remount and occlusal adjustment are completed. It may be necessary to use a soldering iron to lightly heat each guide pin to remove it from the prosthesis (Figs. 3-113 and 3-114).

The final casting can be smoothed with one of several different finishing methods and materials, but continued practice of extreme caution should be taken to protect the gold cylinders from damage during any finishing procedures. Protection caps or brass analogs are placed over the gold cylinders, and the prosthesis is finished and polished using rubber points, wheels, and pumice (Figs. 3-115 and 3-116). A rag wheel with polishing compound is used to give the implant prosthesis its final luster (Fig. 3-117 to 3-119). Soap and water and/or an ultrasonic bath are used to clean residual polishing materials from the prosthesis. The prosthesis is replaced on the master cast, and the interface between the gold cylinders and abutment replicas is checked.

CLINICAL DELIVERY

The patient is to leave out the existing maxillary denture for several hours before the implant prosthesis is inserted, if applicable. Using the usual method the maxillary denture is checked with a pressure indicator paste. A centric relation record is made with both prostheses in position. A laboratory remount is completed. The occlusion is then refined in the mouth using articulating paper and shimstock. The gold screws are tightened with the appropriate torque wrench, and temporary fillings are placed into the screw access holes (Figs. 3-120 to 3-124). The patient then is seen by the hygienist for homecare instructions.

The patient returns to the clinic the following day, and the restorative dentist rechecks the tightness of the screws and discusses any complications that may have occurred overnight with the patient. The patient is scheduled for another recall in 1 week, and the same checks are made. The prosthesis will be permanently seated at the 1-month recall. The patient then is scheduled for recall at 6 months, depending on oral hygiene skills.

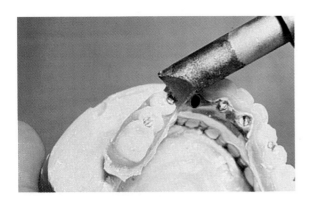

Figure 3-113

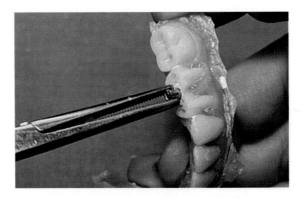

Figure 3-114

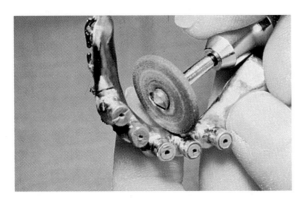

Figure 3-115

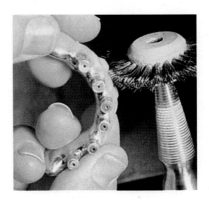

Figure 3-116

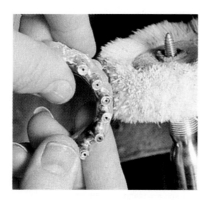

Figure 3-117

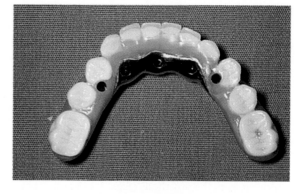

Figure 3-118

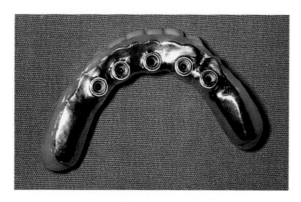

Figure 3-119

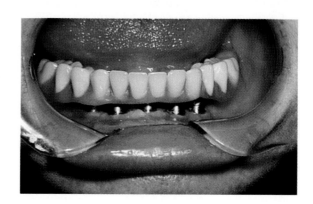

Figure 3-120

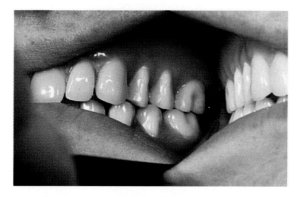

Figure 3-121

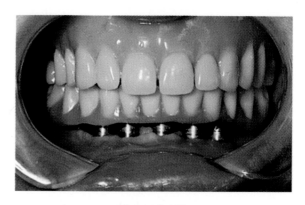

Figure 3-122

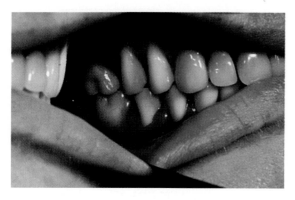

Figure 3-123

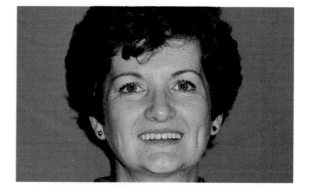

Figure 3-124

Restoring the edentulous maxilla with implant prosthetics is the most challenging area in implant dentistry. Esthetic demands and anatomic considerations make treatment planning, surgery, and laboratory procedures much more complicated than the other types of implant-supported rehabilitation. Teamwork and communication among the different dental disciplines is mandatory in order to ensure an ideal result.

Maxillary teeth are the focal point of the human smile. Proper tooth position establishes the smile line and the amount of tooth and gingival display while providing lip support. The position of maxillary labial bone and soft tissue is equally important for an esthetic facial contour. Advances in surgical techniques allow close to ideal function, hygiene, and esthetics. Implants and the resulting prosthetics are no longer positioned to where resorption has left the remaining bone. Ideal tooth position and facial contour dictate where implants and the underlying bone and soft tissue are positioned. Factors limiting these goals are financial restraints, the skill of the surgeons and restorative dentists, and the desires and expectations of the patient. Treatment planning and teamwork are much more complicated and time consuming, but the results are rewarding.

Procedures to idealize the maxillary anatomy before implant placement may include multiple types of bone grafting in conjunction with orthognathic surgery. Multiple surgical procedures with general anesthesia and some hospital recovery time greatly increases the cost for treatment. The porcelain-fused-to-metal prosthesis with six or more implants is also expensive. Medical and dental insurance rarely cover a great portion of these procedures, and cost may preclude these procedures altogether. Alternative treatment plans are available, which increase function and stop further bone resorption while providing an esthetically acceptable result. These options include several different overdenture designs and the less-expensive hybrid prosthesis using denture teeth and methylmethacrylate resin processed onto a metal framework. Decisions for treatment options need to be made at the initial treatment consultations.

TREATMENT CONSULT

The esthetic desires, functional requirements, and financial realities may dictate the type of implant-retained prosthesis that the patient chooses. When a patient comes to the restorative dentist for an implant consultation, the patient's desires and expectations must be explored. Models of different prosthetic options are shown, including overdentures, porcelain-fused-to-metal prosthesis, and hybrid prosthesis. Photographs of patients who have completed treatment are also useful. The patient's prosthetic problems need to be documented and discussed. An excessive gag reflex may only be eliminated with a palateless prosthesis, such as fixed prosthesis or overdenture with the palate removed. Many female patients have moderate to severe psychologic problems associated with being toothless and its association with old age. Fixed prosthetics, preferable porcelain fused to metal, are desirable for these patients. They will often commit to bone grafting or whatever is necessary to achieve prosthetics that function and look like natural dentition. An overdenture or any removable prosthesis will not be acceptable to patients with this psychologic profile. Frank discussion of patient desires may require several consults. Problems and expectations should be documented and discussed at length. Complications and limitations in treatment outcome should be included in signed consent forms to avoid misunderstandings.

After the patient is interviewed, a clinical examination is completed. The existing dentures are examined for lip support, vertical dimension of occlusion, retention, and esthetics, including height of the smile line. The labial flange thickness of the maxillary denture is measured, and the patient is questioned concerning his or her satisfaction with lip support (Figs 4-1 to 4-4). The distal-most tooth that shows during maximum smile is recorded (Fig. 4-5). Also, a smile line that reveals first or second molars is noted because any implant prosthesis must be treatment planned to extend this far distally.

Fixed prosthetics may require bone grafting and/or placement of implants in the pterygomaxillary region or zygoma to support posterior teeth if the maxillary sinus is large.

Patients who have had recent maxillary extractions may have anatomy favorable for fixed prosthetics without bone grafting. Labial and buccal contour and tissue support need to be evaluated carefully before implant placement to ensure that bone grafting is not needed. The existing maxillary denture may be duplicated if all esthetic and functional parameters are perfect. An ideal trial denture should be made otherwise. The labial and buccal flange of the denture is removed, and the denture is evaluated for facial support. The patient should be involved in the evaluation, and the altered denture should be worn with adhesive for a day or two so the patient has time for evaluation. Lack of support requires labial veneer bone grafting.

SURGICAL EVALUATION

The patient is referred for surgical evaluation. The restorative dentist must relay his findings from the clinical examination and consult the surgeon. Surgical evaluation can then determine if a fixed prosthesis can be made using implants in the existing maxillary anatomy or what augmentation procedures may be necessary to accomplish the type of prosthesis the patient desires. After surgical and prosthetic consults, the restorative dentist and surgeon should meet to review radiographs, pictures, and so on to plan treatment properly.

If orthognathic repositioning of the maxilla is planned, a mounted diagnostic setup of the maxillary denture is required, as well as cephalometric radiographs made with trial denture setup in position. Foil placed against the denture teeth will assist in visualizing incisal edge position radio-graphically compared with existing maxillary bone (see Chapter 5).

CLINICAL AND LABORATORY PROSTHETIC PROCEDURES FOR ALL MAXILLARY FIXED PROSTHETICS
Diagnostic and Surgical Stents

The transitional maxillary denture is used as a guide for the surgical stent. The denture is duplicated and modified. See previously documented fabrication procedures of diagnostic and surgical stents.

TISSUE TREATMENT AFTER SURGERY

In patients who do not have onlay bone grafts, the transitional denture is relieved in the surgical site, and the tissue conditioning material is placed in the denture 7 to 10 days after surgery and the suture removal (Figs. 4-6 and 4-7). The patient occludes lightly while the tissue conditioner sets. After the initial set (approximately 8 to 10 minutes), the denture is placed in a pressure pot at 20 psi for 10 minutes. The tissue conditioner lining is replaced as the patient heals, and the

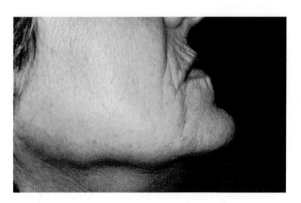

Figure 4-1

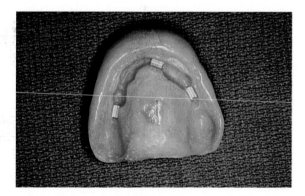

Figure 4-2

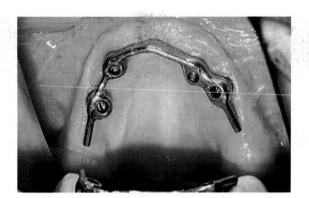

Figure 4-3

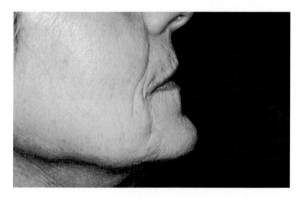

Figure 4-4

denture is relined after complete healing (1½ to 2 months after surgery).

Patients who have had onlay bone grafts are placed on a soft diet for 1 month after surgery, and they do not use a prosthesis. Usually a new denture must be made at this time because the graft will have drastically changed the maxillary morphology.

Tissue treatment material is placed in the relieved prosthesis after second-stage surgery. The healing caps are left on the abutments while the tissue treatment reline is made. The prosthesis has increased retention and stability after this procedure.

STANDARD ABUTMENT

The prosthetic components that are used with the Branemark implant system have a long history of excellence when used in conjunction with patient rehabilitation. The Branemark system components include the titanium implant, which is surgically placed in bone and remains submerged below the mucoperiosteum for 6 to 8 months in the maxilla while the osseointegration occurs. The titanium abutment is placed on the implant during the second surgical procedure (Figs. 4-8 and 4-9). Abutments are available in several lengths to accommodate prosthetic procedures and to allow the abutment to be placed 1 to 2 mm above the soft tissue. The gold screw is used to fix the cylinder, framework, and prosthesis unit to the transmucosal abutments and fixtures. These components are satisfactory for most implant-retained prostheses.

PRELIMINARY IMPRESSION PROCEDURES

Stock edentulous alginate trays are used to make the maxillary impression 10 to 20 days after the abutment surgery (Fig. 4-10). The cast shows the position of the transmucosal abutments in preparation for the custom tray fabrication.

CUSTOM TRAY FABRICATION

The custom tray for the maxillary implant-retained prosthesis is fabricated in the same manner as previously documented for the mandible.

FINAL IMPRESSIONS

The healing caps are removed, and the hexagonal wrench and titanium hemostats are used to check abutment tightness. This procedure should be done at the beginning of every prosthetic appointment. All plaque and calculus are removed,

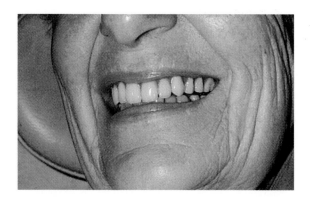

Figure 4-5

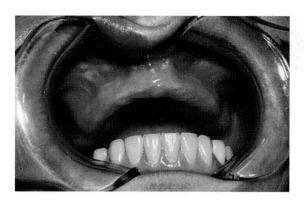

Figure 4-6

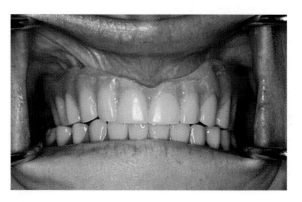

Figure 4-7

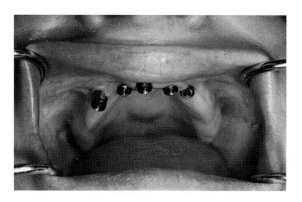

Figure 4-8

and the impression copings are seated (Fig. 4-11). The custom tray is tried in the mouth and is adjusted for path insertion (Fig. 4-12). The window for the tray then is covered with one thickness of baseplate wax, and the edges are sealed with a hot wax spatula (Fig. 4-13). The tray is heated in a water bath and is reseated in the mouth to capture the guide pin relationship (Fig. 4-14). After the adhesive is placed (Fig. 4-15), a medium-viscosity vinyl polysiloxane or other appropriate impression material is mixed according to the manufacturer's directions. A 50 ml syringe and the impression tray are loaded, and the tray is seated in the mouth allowing the guide pins to penetrate the preformed wax holes (Fig. 4-16). The tray is held in position while border molding is completed. After the impression material has set, the guide pins are loosened, and the impression is removed (Fig. 4-17). Laboratory analogs are placed (Fig. 4-18), and the impression is poured in die stone as previously described.

MAXILLOMANDIBULAR RELATIONS

Maxillomandibular relations are recorded using a customized record base and occlusion rim (Figs. 4-19 to 4-21). These are fabricated in a similar fashion as previously described. Gold cylinders or altered impression copings allow the securing of the record base to the abutments for accurate interocclusal records. The wax rims are contoured to establish lip support, incisal edge position, buccal corridor, and midline and ver-

tical dimension of occlusion. Phonetics and other parameters that are employed in conventional denture techniques are also established. Centric relation, eccentric records, a facebow registration, tooth selection, and occlusal scheme are all made by the restorative dentist at this time.

The master cast and the opposing cast are mounted on a semiadjustable articulator. The eccentric records are used for the articulator settings. The master cast is then surveyed, and a full upper denture setup is completed by the laboratory technician.

ANTERIOR AND FULL ESTHETIC TRIAL FITTING

These appointments are used to establish tooth position, esthetics, phonetics, and vertical dimension of occlusion (Figs. 4-22 and 4-23). The transitional denture is used as a guide if the esthetics of the prosthesis are acceptable to the patient and to the restorative dentist. When the esthetics have been approved, the laboratory technician has the guidelines for framework fabrication.

MAXILLARY HYBRID PROSTHESIS

The maxillary hybrid prosthesis was so named because of the combination of metal framework with denture teeth and acrylic. For patients who do not have a high smile line, this option allows a fixed prosthesis at a lower cost to the patient.

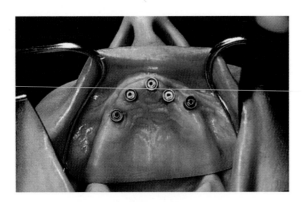

Figure 4-9

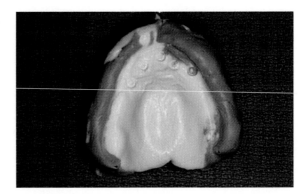

Figure 4-10

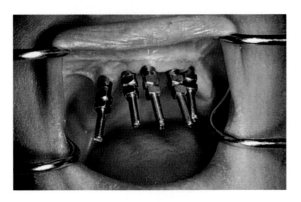

Figure 4-11

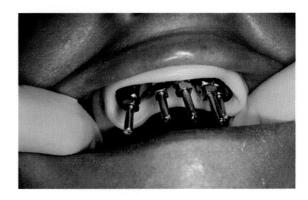

Figure 4-12

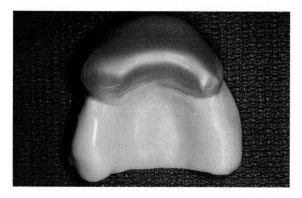

Figure 4-13

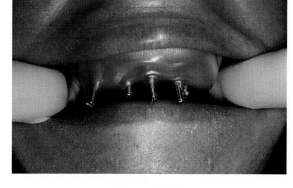

Figure 4-14

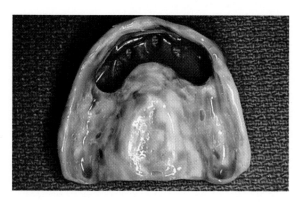

Figure 4-15

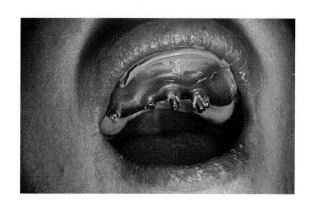

Figure 4-16

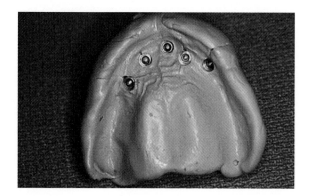

Figure 4-17

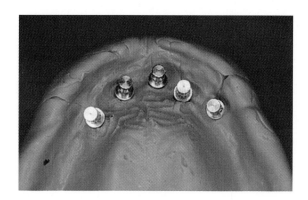

Figure 4-18

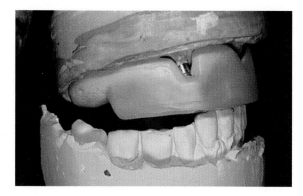

Figure 4-19

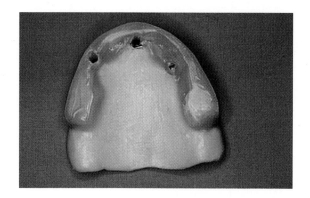

Figure 4-20

The technique is simpler and less expensive than the porcelain-fused-to-metal design but lacks esthetically in some patients because of limits in denture tooth esthetics. If the denture base is visible, esthetics will be compromised compared with pink porcelain available with the porcelain-fused-to-metal prosthesis. Finances dictate the prosthetic choice. The framework design must include adequate room for retentive elements, acrylic, and denture teeth. Processing acrylic and denture teeth onto the frame does not cause framework distortion. Multiple porcelain firings necessary for the porcelain-fused-to-metal framework may cause distortion as a result of porcelain shrinkage. Repair of the broken porcelain after use in the mouth may cause bubbling and explosion of the porcelain because of exposure to saliva. The hybrid prosthesis can be repaired faster and at less cost.

FRAMEWORK FABRICATION

The framework fabrication for the maxillary fixed prosthesis is similar to that for the mandibular prosthesis. The esthetic denture trial fitting is used to establish the relationship of the framework to the final tooth position. The matrix is fabricated in the same manner as previously stated in Chapter

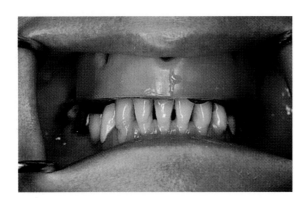

Figure 4-21

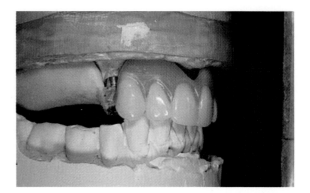

Figure 4-22

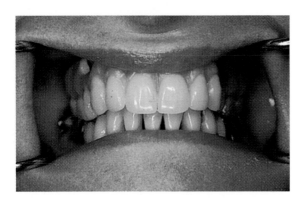

Figure 4-23

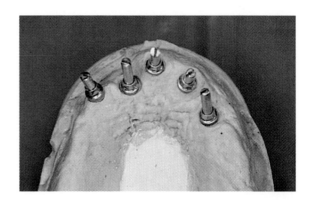

Figure 4-24

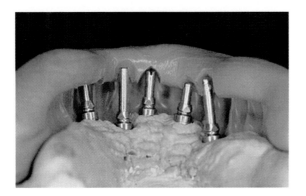

Figure 4-25

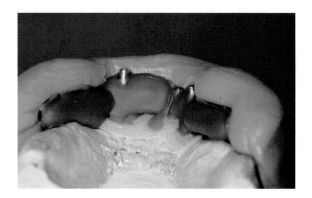

Figure 4-26

3. The gold cylinders are placed on the master cast with guide pins (Fig. 4-24). The master cast is blocked out with compound, the guide pins are lubricated, and the matrix is reoriented to the master cast and held in place with sticky wax (Fig. 4-25). The matrix is filled with molten inlay wax and is allowed to solidify (Fig 4-26). The matrix is removed, and the full contoured waxing is completed (Fig. 4-27). Proper contours must be incorporated into the framework design of the implant prosthesis. Ideally, convex surfaces are more desirable, allowing access for plaque removal. Cutback is performed, and retention is provided for final processing of the denture base resin and for placement of teeth (Fig. 4-28). The wax pattern is indirectly sprued, invested, cast, reclaimed, and replaced on the master cast for fit verification (Figs. 4-29 to 4-31).

CLINICAL—FRAMEWORK TRIAL FITTING

The healing caps are removed, the abutments are cleaned and tightened, and the framework is seated passively with guide pins or gold screws (Figs. 4-32 and 4-33). Each abutment framework interface is checked circumferentially for

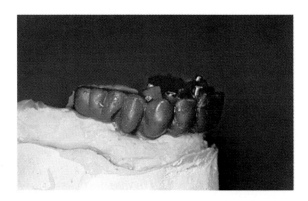

Figure 4-27

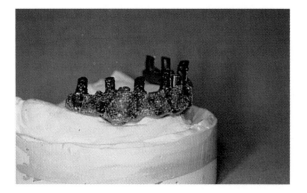

Figure 4-28

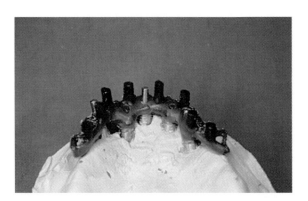

Figure 4-29

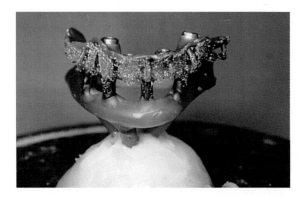

Figure 4-30

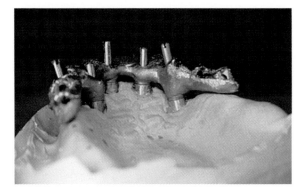

Figure 4-31

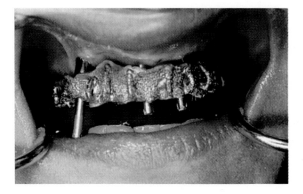

Figure 4-32

intimacy of fit. Mirror views are used for verification of the palatal interface. Any discrepancy in the interface requires that the framework be sectioned, reverifying fit and solder indexing as seen previously in Chapter 3.

The framework fit is reverified if soldering was necessary. Another indication that the framework may be inaccurate occurs when the patient experiences sensitivity during the tightening of the screws. If sensitivity persists during several attempts at sequential slow tightening of the prosthetic screws, then the framework in the area of the sensitive

implant must be sectioned, and a new solder index must be made.

FULL ESTHETIC TRIAL FITTING

The matrix used for framework waxing is used as a guide for resetting teeth on the frame. Esthetics and other parameters are verified again, and a centric relation record is made (Fig. 4-34). Adjustable mirrors may be useful in verifying esthetics. Lateral views are beneficial for patient verification of lip and tissue support. A friend or relative may be helpful at the

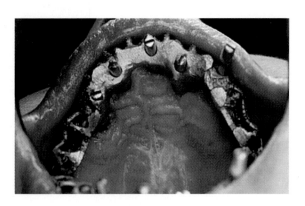

Figure 4-33

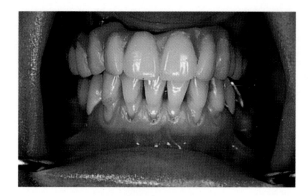

Figure 4-34

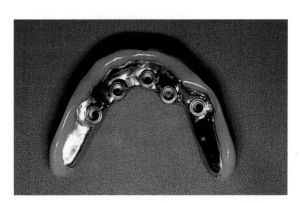

Figure 4-35

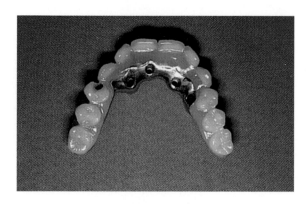

Figure 4-36

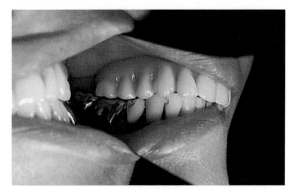

Figure 4-37

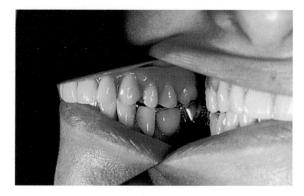

Figure 4-38

full tooth arrangement appointment when the patient makes a final decision about the esthetics of the arrangement.

PROCESSING AND FINISHING

The laboratory processing and finishing procedures are performed for the maxillary implant prosthesis in the same manner as previously documented in Chapter 3 for the mandible. The finished prosthesis is ready for delivery to the patient (Figs. 4-35 and 4-36).

CLINICAL DELIVERY

The healing caps are removed, the abutments are cleaned and tightened, and the prosthesis is seated (Figs. 4-37 to 4-41). The gold screws are sequentially tightened using the torque wrench for final tightness (Fig. 4-42). Occlusion is checked with occlusal ribbon and shimstock. If occlusal discrepancies have occurred during framework processing, a laboratory remount will be required. Cotton pellets and a temporary filling material are placed in the screw access holes. The patient then is seen by the hygienist for home care instructions and hygiene armamentarium. The patient is scheduled for recalls as described previously. Final filling is done as previously described.

PORCELAIN-FUSED-TO-METAL PROSTHESIS

The porcelain-fused-to-metal prosthesis is the restoration of choice for restoring the maxilla for optimum esthetics and most closely mimics natural dentition. A diagnostic setup of the teeth is tried in the patient's mouth to verify esthetics, and a matrix of this setup is used as a guide for placing porcelain on the metal framework (Fig. 4-43). A high smile line may cause esthetic and hygiene compromise if the hybrid prosthesis is used (Figs. 4-44 and 4-45). Modified ridge lap pontics using a porcelain-fused-to-metal design may be more esthetic and accessible for cleaning. The patient seen in Figs. 4-44 and 4-45 was able to clean more effectively while avoiding denture base display by changing to a porcelain-fused-to-metal prosthesis (Figs. 4-46 and 4-47).

The pioneering Swedish implant teams used porcelain-fused-to-metal restorations as well as resin veneering systems. They found a higher incidence of implant loss with the porcelain-fused-to-metal prosthesis and therefore recommended using the resin systems for esthetic veneers. A dampening effect from the resin during mastication and parafunctional activities was believed to be a positive influence of preserving osseointegration, although it was not

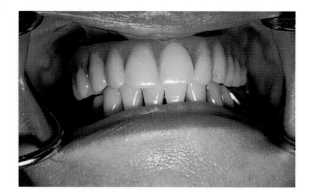

Figure 4-39

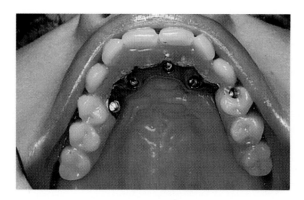

Figure 4-40

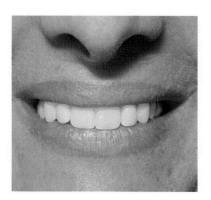

Figure 4-41

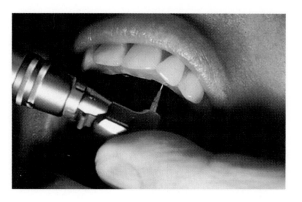

Figure 4-42

scientifically proven. Resin is much less esthetic than porcelain.

A prosthetic design has been developed that incorporates the advantages of both materials. The framework has porcelain applied on the buccal surface to a 1 mm metal finish line on the palatal slope of the buccal cusps (Figs. 4-48 and 4-49). Light-cured composite is used on the occlusal surface of the posterior teeth in all areas of occlusal contact. Therefore the esthetics of the porcelain are combined with the dampening effect and wear pattern of the composite resin (Fig. 4-50).

Impression technique, maxillomandibular relations, and trial fitting appointments for the porcelain-fused-to-metal prosthesis are the same as those described earlier in this chapter. Because of the implant position and lack of intermaxillary space, the UCLA-type abutment was used for this patient (see Chapter 6 for details).

A matrix of the trial setup is made. Gold cylinders with guide pins are placed as previously described. Wax is flowed from an eyedropper into the matrix around the guide pins and the gold cylinders. The waxing is carved and refined around the gold cylinders. Buccal and incisal areas are cut

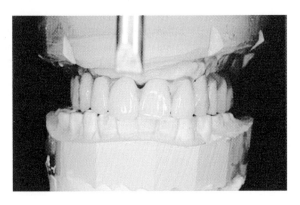

Figure 4-43

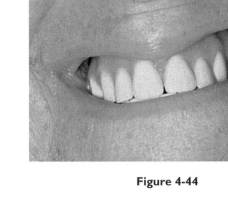

Figure 4-44

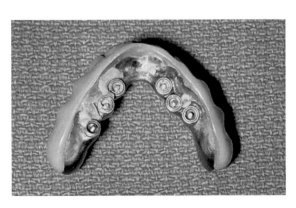

Figure 4-45

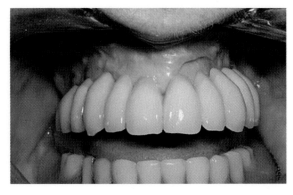

Figure 4-46

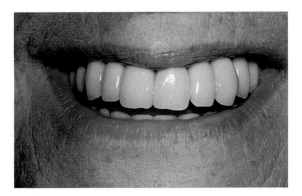

Figure 4-47

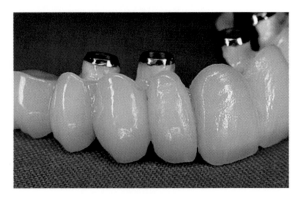

Figure 4-48

back 1.5 to 2 mm for porcelain application (Fig. 4-51). A 1 mm finish line is maintained on the palatal slope of the buccal cusps (Fig. 4-52). At least 2 mm of wax is cut back (palatal to the finish line) for light-cured resin application. Plastic retentive beads and undercuts are placed for composite retention. Investing, casting, and reclaiming are described in Chapter 3.

The framework is placed on the implants and checked for accurate implant-framework interface. All subgingival implant-framework interfaces, such as UCLA or EsthetiCone abutments, require radiographic verification of fit since visual inspection is impossible (Fig. 4-53). Inaccurate interface or pain experienced by the patient when the abutment screws are tightened requires framework sectioning and solder index (Figs. 4-54 and 4-55).

The metal framework is finished to receive the porcelain application. Opaque is applied and fired to the frame (Fig. 4-56). A full porcelain contour is designed, and the first bake is completed (Fig. 4-57). Adjustments are made as necessary, with anatomic contours as designed in the provisional set-up. The bisque trial fitting is returned for an esthetic evaluation and fitting (Fig. 4-58).

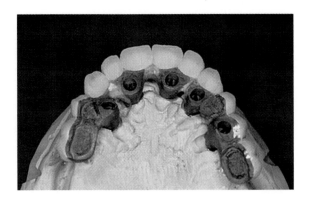

Figure 4-49

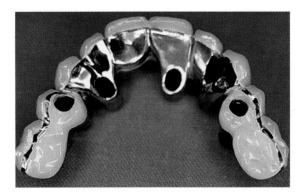

Figure 4-50

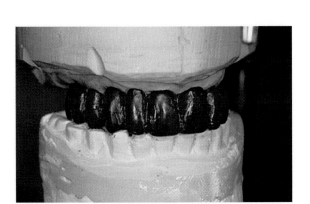

Figure 4-51

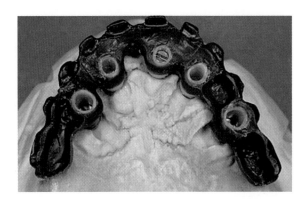

Figure 4-52

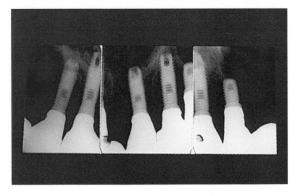

Figure 4-53

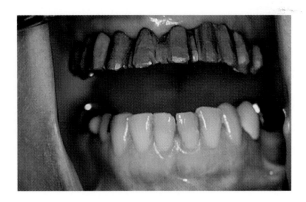

Figure 4-54

The abutments are removed, and the prosthesis is seated. The implant or abutment-framework interface is checked for accuracy. Lip support, incisal edge position, porcelain contours, and midline are evaluated and modified. The porcelain value, hue, and chroma are evaluated for modification and staining. When the porcelain contours and esthetics have been approved, the prosthesis is ready for posterior composite placement. Centric relation records are made, and the prosthesis is removed. The abutments are placed on the implants and tightened.

When the bisqued prosthesis is returned to the laboratory, esthetic corrections are made and the prosthesis is glazed and polished. Protective measures (as previously documented) should be continually followed, thereby preventing damage to the interface surfaces (Fig. 4-59). The occlusal retentive areas that will receive the composite are metal treated, and microfilled composite is processed to the framework. The completed prosthesis is polished and ready for delivery to the patient (Fig. 4-60).

The patient in Figs. 4-61 and 4-62 had severe anterior maxillary bone resorption from wearing a complete denture along with mandibular natural dentition. A nasal inlay bone graft was harvested from below the apices of the mandibular natural dentition and placed into the floor of the nose.

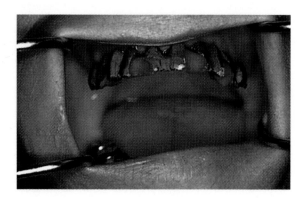

Figure 4-55

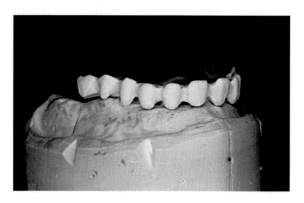

Figure 4-56

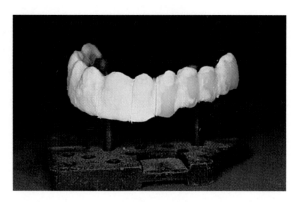

Figure 4-57

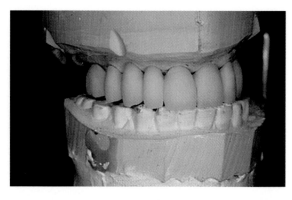

Figure 4-58

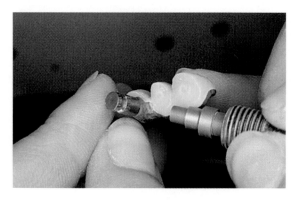

Figure 4-59

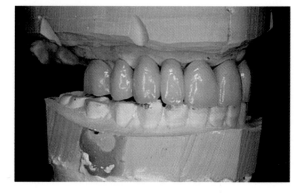

Figure 4-60

The maxillary combination prosthesis is seated. The interfaces are checked for accuracy radiographically. Occlusal ribbon and shimstock are used to perfect the occlusion. A laboratory remount may be used for occlusal adjustment also. After the prosthesis is polished, it is seated, and the gold screws are tightened using the torque wrench. Temporary fillings are placed in the screw access holes (Figs. 4-63 to 4-70).

SPARK EROSION PROSTHESIS

Long-term edentulism, trauma, or congenital defect may leave maxillary anatomy unfavorable for an ideal maxillary fixed prosthesis. Many edentulous patients have used the labial flange of the maxillary denture to restore labial contours. Bone grafting to augment these contours may not be financially feasible, or the patient may elect to have the prosthetics restore contour while being removable for hygiene.

The spark erosion prosthesis is composed of a screw-retained substructure with custom slots and latch receptacles, which allows for securing of a second section with a metal framework with either denture teeth or a porcelain-fused-to-metal design, which also contains a labial flange for lip support. The primary substructure attaches to the abutments. The secondary section of the prosthesis attaches to the primary unit with parallel slots and is latched in place. These sections act as a fixed prosthesis functionally while allowing removal for hygiene of the secondary unit. Most of the palate is not covered by prosthesis.

Clinical procedures involve initial impressions after abutment surgery. A custom tray is used to make a fixture level impression. A trial denture setup without a labial flange is completed establishing tooth position, vertical dimension of occlusion, phonetics, and esthetics in the usual fashion (Fig. 4-71). The trial denture setup is used to select abutments and to establish labial support. The final impression is made in the usual fashion after placement of abutments. The master cast is mounted against the mandibular arch using the finished trial denture setup. The laboratory fabricates the substructure framework, which is evaluated for fit clinically as previously described for other implant frameworks (Figs. 4-72 and 4-73). Sectioning and soldering is completed as needed until passive fit is attained between abutments and the substructure framework. The laboratory technician fabricates the superstructure framework using a spark erosion technique. Guide slots and latches are incorporated into the metal framework (see Fig. 4-72). Sufficient cutback in the

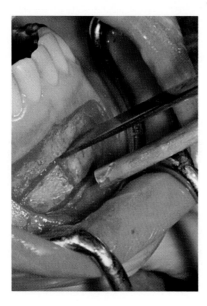

Figure 4-61

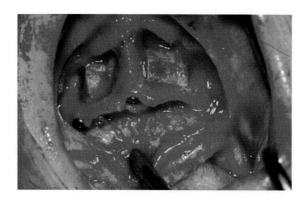

Figure 4-62

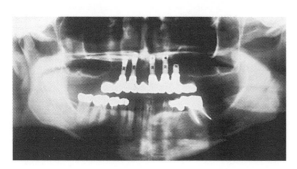

Figure 4-63

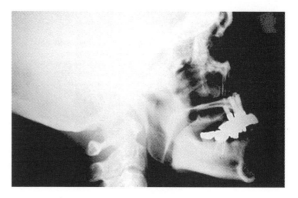

Figure 4-64

secondary unit is completed to allow addition of denture teeth and acrylic or to allow porcelain application. The complete laboratory technique for fabricating both sections of the spark erosion prosthesis is beyond the scope of this text. The completed prosthesis is seen in Figs. 4-74 to 4-81.

BONE GRAFTING THE MAXILLA

When evaluating the maxilla for prosthetic options, inadequate tissue contours for facial support or inadequate bone for a sufficient number of implants may preclude fabricating a fixed prosthesis. A patient's strong desire for the fixed prosthetic option and psychologic aversion to a removable pros-

thesis are indications for augmentation using autogenous bone grafts. The bony deficits dictate the size and harvest site for the graft (Fig. 4-82 and 4-83).

Full Onlay Bone Graft

The full onlay bone graft ad modem Branemark is indicated for patients with extreme resorption of the maxilla or congenital or traumatic defects. Two major surgical sites are involved: the iliac crest and the maxilla. The procedure requires general anesthesia and up to 5 days of hospitalization. Six to eight implants are normally placed. No maxillary interim denture wear is allowed for up to 5 weeks, depend-

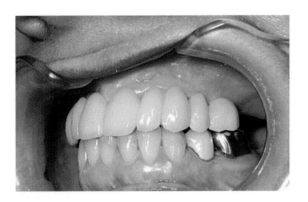

Figure 4-65

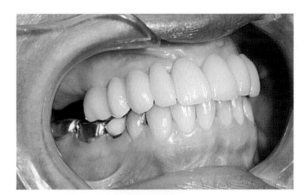

Figure 4-66

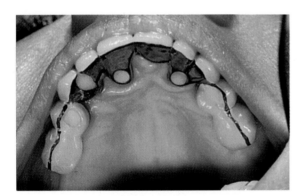

Figure 4-67

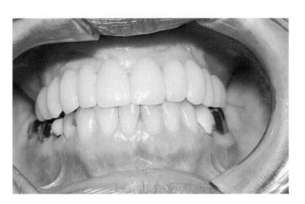

Figure 4-68

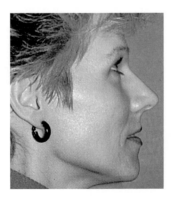

Figure 4-69

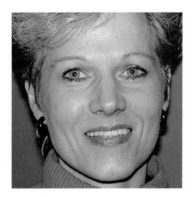

Figure 4-70

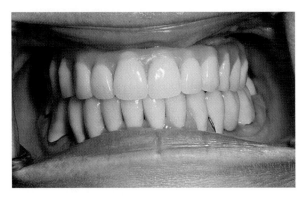

Figure 4-71

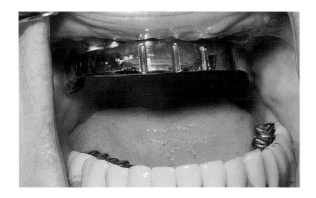

Figure 4-72

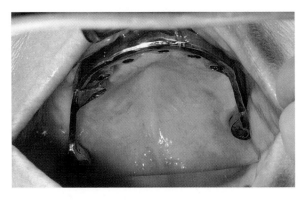

Figure 4-73

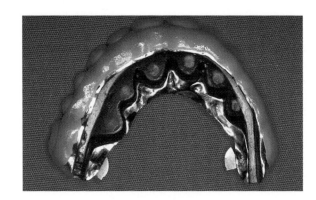

Figure 4-74

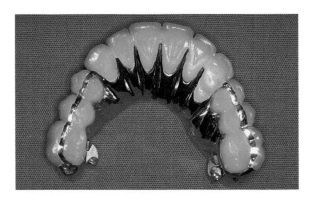

Figure 4-75

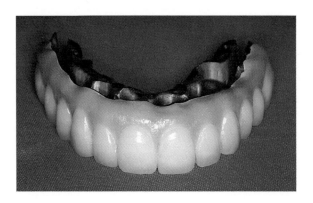

Figure 4-76

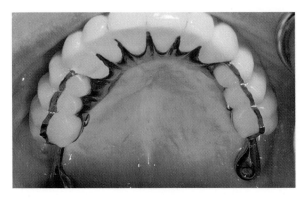

Figure 4-77

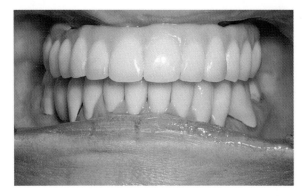

Figure 4-78

ing on the surgeon's wishes. The change in maxillary morphology after grafting requires that a new interim denture be made. The patient is placed on a soft diet for 6 to 9 months before abutment surgery. The patient shown in Fig. 4-84 was adamant about receiving a fixed maxillary prosthesis. A full onlay bone graft was placed and secured with six implants. In addition, implants were placed bilaterally in the pterygomaxillary regions. A fixed prosthesis was completed (Fig. 4-85 to 4-89) using pink porcelain applied gingival to the teeth for labial support. Though not apparent in Figs. 4-85 to 4-87, all areas of the prosthesis were cleanable, and the patient's home care was impeccable.

The surgical technique with onlay grafting involves anchoring of the graft to the residual maxillary bone. Implant position is often palatal to where the natural dentition originally was. The prosthesis will, therefore, be cantilevered to the anterior. Speech is often initially compromised, and access for hygiene may be difficult.

In most patients, speech returns to normal within 1 to 6 months. Individual implant survival and overall prosthetic success is high.

Chapter 5 presents a surgical technique that repositions the maxilla down and forward. This compensates for the maxillary resorption pattern.

PTERYGOMAXILLARY IMPLANTS

Bone located in the maxillary posterior is poor in quality and volume. The maxillary sinus is often large in patients who have been edentulous for long periods of time. Implants are often necessary in the posterior maxilla to support prosthetic extensions necessary for including first and second molars on the prosthesis. Bone grafting to the sinus adds to the cost and morbidity to implant rehabilitation. Distal and slightly medial to the tuberosity, adequate bone is formed by the perpendicular plate and pyramidal process of the palatine bone and the pterygoid process of the sphenoid. This region, referred to as the *pterygomaxillary region*, contains a dense cortical bone and is ideal for implant replacement. Implants placed bilaterally in this area can provide distal anchorage for a fixed prosthesis. This anchorage eliminates the need for a cantilever and allows first and second molars to be placed on the prosthesis. Elimination of the cantilever allows for more even distribution of force to each implant, which should reduce complications such as component loosening and breakage. Additional posterior teeth provide better mastication. Esthetics are improved for patients who display posterior teeth. Eliminating the need for bone grafting decreases the time for treatment and greatly decreases expenses.

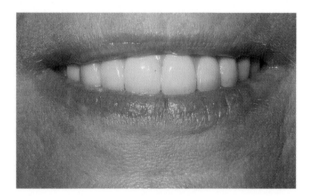

Figure 4-79

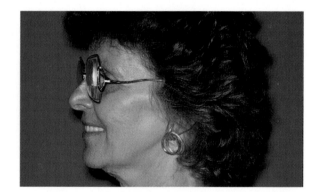

Figure 4-80

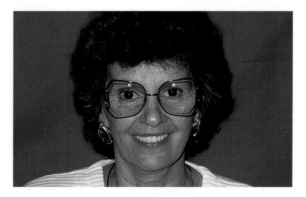

Figure 4-81

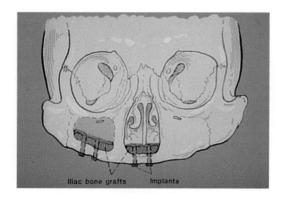

Figure 4-82

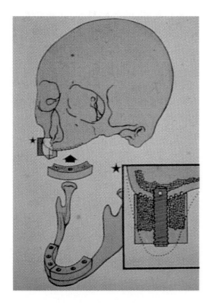

Figure 4-83

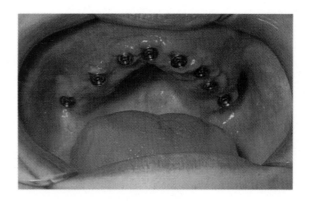

Figure 4-84

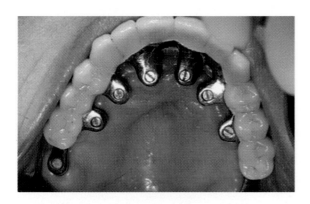

Figure 4-85

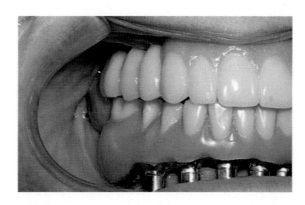

Figure 4-86

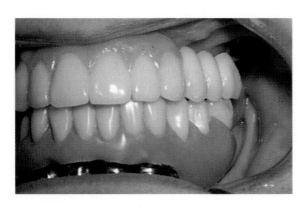

Figure 4-87

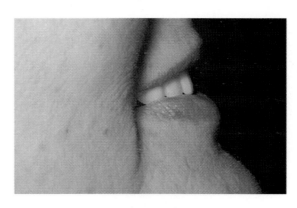

Figure 4-88

The patient in Figs. 4-90 to 4-97 desired a fixed prosthesis. She was prepared to have sinus inlay grafting or onlay grafting if necessary to ensure enough implants for a fixed prosthesis. Large maxillary sinuses precluded implant placement in the alveolus posterior to the first bicuspid. A high smile line displayed first molars (see Fig. 4-97). Surgical exploration revealed solid bone in the pterygomaxillary region, and implants were placed bilaterally with good initial anchorage. Prosthetics were completed in the usual fashion. Access for placement of components was difficult. The mandibular implant-supported prosthesis was removed to allow room for final impressions.

NASAL INLAY BONE GRAFT

Patients with mandibular anterior teeth who are edentulous in the maxilla often have more severe bone loss in the anterior maxilla. Nasal inlay grafting is indicated in this situation. Bone may be harvested from the iliac crest or from the anterior mandible, if available (see Figs. 4-61 and 4-62). The remaining prosthetic procedures for this patient are seen in Figs. 4-48 to 4-68.

Chapter 5 discusses additional bone grafting techniques, including inlay grafting in combination with orthognathic surgery. Labial veneer grafting is discussed as well.

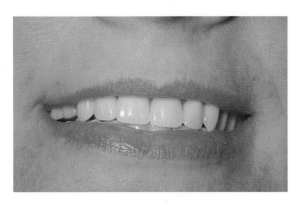

Figure 4-89

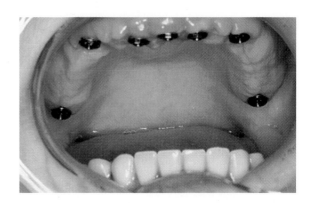

Figure 4-90

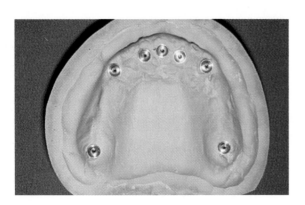

Figure 4-91

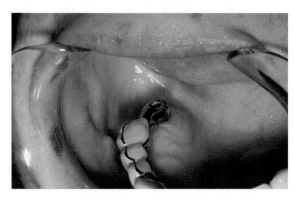

Figure 4-92

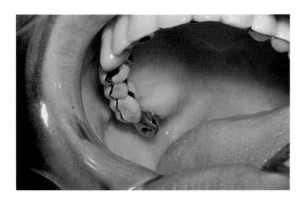

Figure 4-93

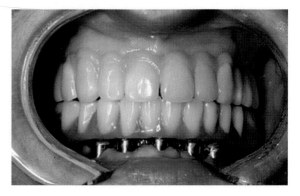

Figure 4-94

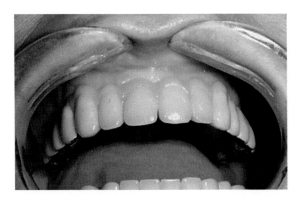

Figure 4-95

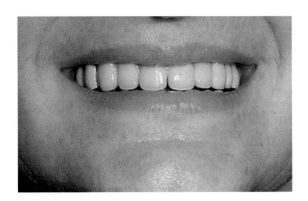

Figure 4-96

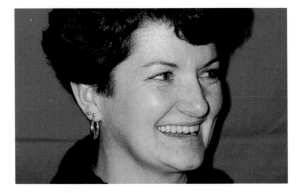

Figure 4-97

Treatment Planning and Surgical Considerations for Bone-Grafted Maxilla

Clark O. Taylor
Patrick J. Stevens

Treatment of the atrophic edentulous maxilla has long represented a significant challenge to the reconstructive surgeon. Early loss of secondary dentition sets in motion a chain of events that ultimately leads to deterioration of masticatory function and facial esthetics. Use of traditional denture prostheses accelerates this process and causes a variety of soft and hard tissue changes.[1] The maxilla is somewhat more resistant to resorption than the mandible and typically resorbs at a rate 1/4 to 1/5 that of the lower jaw.[2,3] Because ridge resorption is chronic and progressive, it results in soft tissue, functional, psychologic, social, and facial aesthetic problems. Therefore any reconstructive efforts directed at the atrophic edentulous maxilla should consider all of the above noted affected parameters. With proper treatment planning, restoration and improvement in most, if not all, of the affected parameters noted above are possible, leading to a more ideal treatment end point and a more satisfied patient population.

EXAMINATION AND TREATMENT PLANNING

Examination and treatment planning may be subdivided into three areas.

1. An overall clinical assessment of facial proportions and contours is made.
2. Soft tissue changes associated with the aging face and edentulism are evaluated. This includes the mandibular genial angle and mandibular inferior border contours as well as an assessment of the chin and submental region. The presence of the midfacial soft tissue aesthetics affected by maxillary edentulism specifically would include addressing of the nasolabial angle and nasal tip ptosis, as well as an assessment of the nasolabial furrows. As the osseous resorption progresses, an increasing acuteness of the nasolabial angle with secondary nasal tip ptosis, as well as a loss of lip support, leads to an accentuation of the aging face syndrome.
3. An intraoral evaluation of jaw relationship, vestibular depth, residual maxillary ridge form, and the condition of keratinized and nonkeratinized tissue is made. It is important to keep in mind that, as bimaxillary resorption occurs, a pseudo-class III ridge relationship naturally

occurs. If the patient exhibited a class III occlusal relationship in a dentate state, the class III edentulous jaw relationship can become extremely severe. The radiographic evaluation includes a panoramic film, which allows evaluation of residual maxillary alveolus as well as position and proximity of the nasal and sinus cavities. A lateral cephalogram is obtained in all patients with a maxillary prosthesis (permanent or temporary wax try-in), which exhibits proper vertical dimension and ideal or a desired final maxillary incisal position. It is extremely important that the prosthetic dentist establish a precise maxillary incisal position at this point in the treatment planning because this is the treatment end point for all implant-supported reconstruction. Using a lateral cephalogram, precise measurements may be made to determine the discrepancy between the residual maxillary bony alveolus and the desired maxillary incisal position.

Most authors today promote the use of a removable implant-supported prosthesis for maxillary reconstruction. This treatment is used because of the necessity for cantilevering to establish ideal incisal position and because of hygiene and phonetic problems associated with maxillary fixed prosthetics. Because of the relative lack of variability in maxillary incisor position, if a fixed prosthesis is desired as the treatment end point, this can only be accomplished by osseous reconstruction with a degree of accuracy allowing normal emergent anatomy with the implant-supported anterior dental prosthetic segments. Traditional onlay techniques are notoriously inaccurate because of the variable resorption and remodeling that takes place, as well as the lack of precise preoperative treatment planning. The use of precise maxillary repositioning via LeFort I osteotomy with interpositional grafting, and in some cases veneer onlay grafting, allows precise repositioning with minimal alteration in maxillary ridge form. The patient then becomes a candidate for a fixed prosthesis as all of the previously noted problems are potentially eliminated. In addition, the patient is able to wear a removable maxillary prosthesis in the immediate postoperative period because the crestal ridge anatomy is not significantly altered. Patient acceptance of fixed prosthetics is much higher because the use of a removable prosthesis is still, in the mind of the patient, a "denture." The self-confidence and functional improvement with fixed prosthesis is unmatched, and the improvement in soft tissue contour using LeFort I repositioning is highly desirable and unmatched with onlay grafting techniques.

SURGICAL TREATMENT

Using a LeFort I osteotomy, the maxilla is downfractured and repositioned using osseous reference marks and the surgical stent. The surgical stent is articulated with a lower denture, which is secured with circummandibular wires to the edentulous mandible or to natural dentition if present. In addition, maxillary incisal tooth display can be ascertained intraoperatively and confirmed. The implants may be placed simultaneously if 3 to 4 mm of residual alveolus is present to support the implants or inserted in a staged fashion 5 months after the grafting procedure. The maxilla itself is reconstructed using sinus inlay grafts after removal of all sinus mucosa. The sinus inlay grafts are secured with 2 mm bone screws or simultaneously placed implants using the prefabricated surgical stent to ensure adequate and precise axial inclination of the implants. The nasal floor is reconstructed using a sandwiched inlay graft, secured once again by either intraosseous 2 mm screws or simultaneously placed implants. Finally, veneer grafts are placed as indicated and secured with screws. All of the necessary autogenous bone is obtained from the anterior iliac crest, and in cases of upper and lower jaw reconstructions, occasional bilateral anterior iliac crests are used. The posterior ilium is also used in certain situations; however, the contours of the corticocancellous blocks are less ideal than those obtained from the anterior ilium.

Once the maxilla is repositioned and the interpositional grafts are placed, the maxilla is rigidly fixated using 1.5 mm plates and screws. The intraosseous gaps of the lateral maxillary wall are filled with autogenous bone. The interim prosthesis is either inserted immediately with a palatal screw or relieved with a soft tissue adhesive liner in 10 to 14 days. If immediate insertion with a palatal screw is elected, great care must be taken to ensure that no pressure points exist over the palatal mucosa because this represents the sole blood supply to the pedicle maxillary segment. If delayed implant insertion

is chosen, it is performed between 5 and 6 months postoperatively using the same surgical stent. The implants, if placed simultaneously, are exposed in 7 to 9 months, and if inserted in a staged fashion, they are allowed to integrate for 4 months. Any necessary soft tissue procedures are performed after the stage II operation, including keratinized tissue grafts. Associated soft tissue cosmetic procedures, which are frequently used in this group of patients (e.g., face lift [rhytidectomy], eye lift [blepharoplasty], and rhinoplasty), are conveniently performed at the stage II procedure. The final prosthesis is a porcelain-fused-to-metal prosthesis that exhibits ideal emergence profiles, provided that proper preoperative treatment planning and intraoperative execution have occurred. With accurate presurgical planning and precise operative technique, the problems traditionally associated with fixed maxillary implant-supported bridges are eliminated. Phonetic problems, adverse biomechanical factors such as cantilevering, and hygiene problems caused by food entrapment are extremely rare. The patient's acceptance of the ultimate prosthesis is extremely satisfying, and to date, the prostheses have functioned well without prosthetic-induced problems. This technique has been used for the past 10 years.

Fig. 5-1 shows an extremely resorbed maxilla restored with onlay grafting and a fixed prosthesis. The extreme distance from the abutments to the incisal edge position with resultant long cantilever is a disadvantage of the onlay graft technique. This patient adapted her speech with no residual problems and is able to clean the prosthesis with little difficulty. The patient seen in Fig. 5-2 had a traditional hybrid prosthesis in the mandible with extreme resorption in the maxilla (Fig. 5-3). Foil was placed on the denture teeth, and the lateral cephalometric film was used to measure the amount of advancement and downgrafting necessary to restore the maxilla. Mounted diagnostic casts were used for model surgery (Fig. 5-4). The maxillary cast was dropped and advanced, held in position with plaster (Fig. 5-5). A surgical template was made to help position the maxilla. After LeFort procedures, the template is used to verify maxillary position (Fig. 5-6). Calipers are used with reference marks as scored in the maxilla to verify maxillary position (Fig. 5-7).

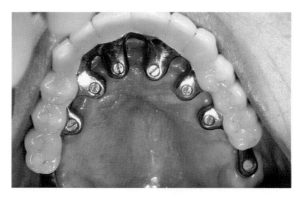

Figure 5-1

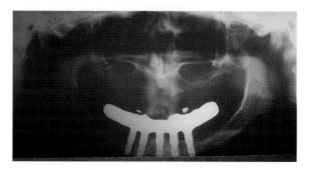

Figure 5-2

Labial veneer grafting is often necessary for labial support (Fig. 5-8). This information is communicated to the surgeon after fabricating the treatment denture with ideal labial support. The flange thickness is measured. A postgrafting panorex shows the stabilized graft (Figs. 5-9 and 5-10). After 5 months, a surgical template was used to guide implant placement (Fig. 5-11). A panorex and lateral cephalometric radiograph show implants in position (Figs. 5-12 and 5-13).

The finished porcelain-fused-to-metal prosthesis is seen from an occlusal view (Fig. 5-14). Notice the screw access position exiting through the cingulum of the anterior teeth and the occlusal surface of the posterior teeth. A frontal view of the porcelain-fused-to-metal prosthesis is shown in Fig. 5-15. The mandibular implant prosthesis will be reset because of occlusal wear and straining from 6 years of use.

Hopeless remaining natural dentition is seen in Fig. 5-16. A lateral cephalometric radiograph shows ideal incisor position in relation to the maxillary bone (Fig. 5-17). Fig. 5-18 shows the finished surgical template prosthesis used with foil for a lateral cephalometric radiograph.

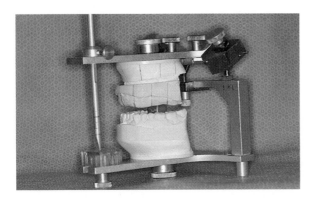

Figure 5-3

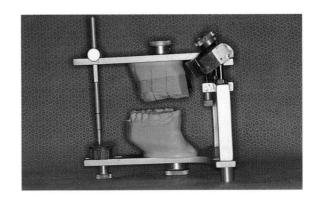

Figure 5-4

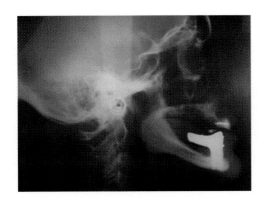

Figure 5-5

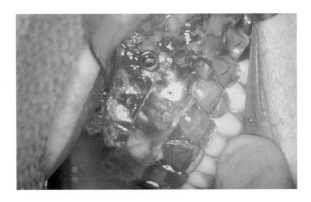

Figure 5-6

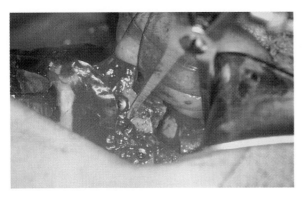

Figure 5-7

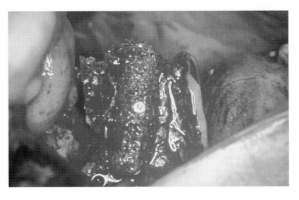

Figure 5-8

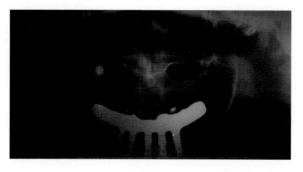

Figure 5-9

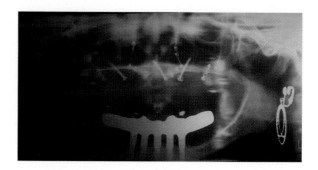

Figure 5-10

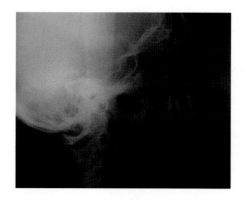

Figure 5-11

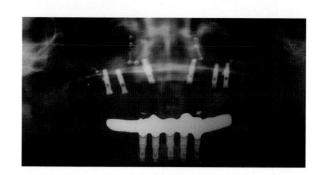

Figure 5-12

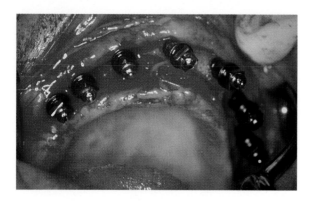

Figure 5-13

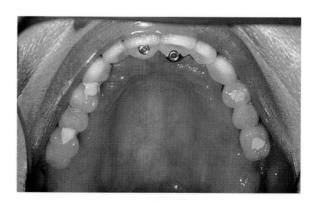

Figure 5-14

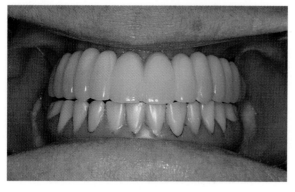

Figure 5-15

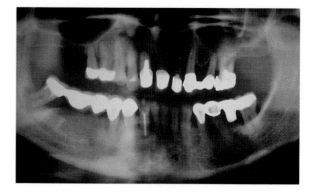

Figure 5-16

PROSTHETIC PREPARATION FOR MAXILLARY LEFORT I OSTEOTOMY WITH INTERPOSITIONAL AND LABIAL VENEER GRAFTING

A maxillary denture is fabricated with the precise incisor tooth position at the proper vertical dimension of occlusion. The position of the maxillary incisors determines the amount of maxillary advancement and the inferior position of the maxilla after interpositional bone grafting. Although a wax trial denture may be acceptable, a processed denture prevents tooth dislodgement from the wax. The denture is mounted at the proper vertical dimension against the lower cast on a semiadjustable articulator. Vaseline is placed between the mounting plaster and the stone supporting the maxillary prosthesis to allow ease of separation during model surgery.

Before model surgery, a putty or plaster matrix is made relating the ideal position of the maxillary teeth to the mandibular arch. This matrix can be used for fabricating a transitional maxillary denture because the relationship between the tooth position and the lower cast is preserved and can be used to facilitate, quickly making the transitional maxillary denture after sufficient healing.

Close communication between the oral surgeon and prosthodontist is mandatory to ensure that the maxilla is moved to the correct position at the correct vertical dimension while allowing room for prosthetic components, framework, and porcelain.

The transitional denture can be duplicated in a clear acrylic to provide a surgical stent to guide implant position (see Fig. 5-18). Adequate labial support is extremely important to allow proper lip support and access for hygiene. The maxilla can be restored to preextraction conformation with proper planning and technique. The fixed prosthesis will be easier to clean, and speech adaptation occurs much faster compared with the onlay bone grafting method.

The mandibular hybrid prosthesis was fabricated first on seven implants. The maxillary surgical template is shown on the lateral cephalometric film in Fig. 5-19. The incisal edge position was used to measure remaining maxillary bone and determine the distance to advance and drop the maxilla to put implants in an ideal position existing from the angulum area of the central lateral incisors and cuspids. Posterior exit holes were planned for the central fossa of selected posterior teeth. After downfracture of the maxilla, implants are seen in the maxillary bone (Figs. 5-20 and 5-21). Occlusal and frontal photographs show abutment position (Figs. 5-22 and 5-23). Seventeen-degree angulated abutments were used on the four anterior implants, placing the screw access holes directly through the angulums of teeth 6, 8, 9, and 11 (Fig. 5-24). Standard abutments were used on the four posterior implants placing the screw access holes through the occlusal surface of

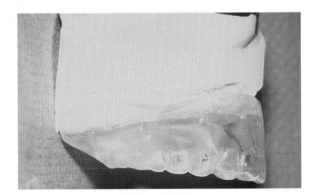

Figure 5-17

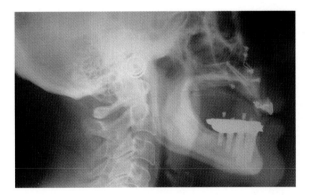

Figure 5-18

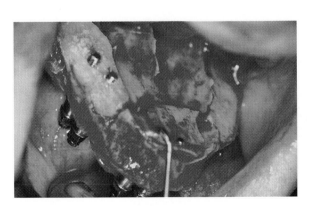

Figure 5-19

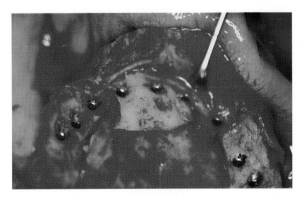

Figure 5-20

teeth 2, 3, 14, and 15. By carefully planning the maxillary and mandibular rehabilitation with communication between the surgeon and prosthodontist and the use of surgical stents, diagnostic setups, and radiographs study casts with model surgery, absolutely perfect implant position was obtained. The patient's adaptation for speech and the ability to chew and clean was immediate. Right and left lateral photographs show the teeth in occlusion with adequate space for hygiene (Figs. 5-25 and 5-26). Other clinical views are seen in Figs. 5-27 to 5-29, showing tooth display and ideal lip support resulting from ideal position and labial veneer grafting.

References

1. Tallgren A: The continuing reduction of the alveolar ridges in complete denture wearers: a mixed longitudinal study covering 25 years. *J Prosthet Dent*, 28:2, 1972.
2. Atwood DA: Some clinical factors related to the rate of resorption of residual ridges. *J Prosthet Dent*, 12:3, 1962.
3. Atwood DA: Reduction of residual ridges: a major oral disease entity. *J Prosthet Dent*, 26:3, 1971.

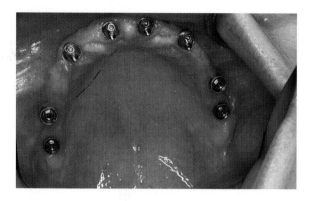

Figure 5-21

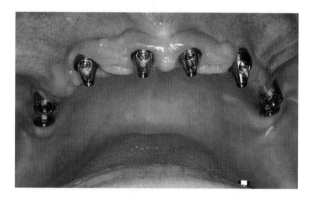

Figure 5-22

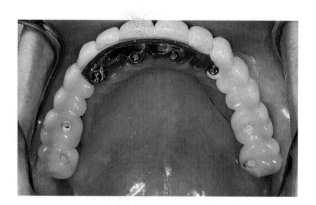

Figure 5-23

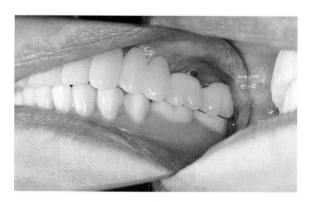

Figure 5-24

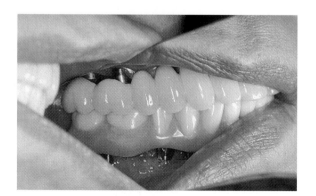

Figure 5-25

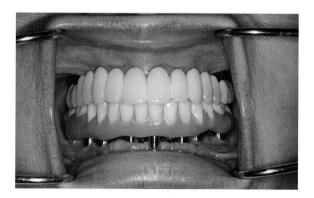

Figure 5-26

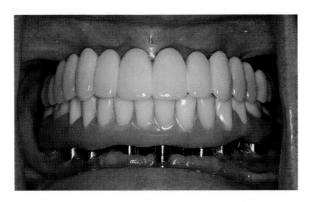

Figure 5-27

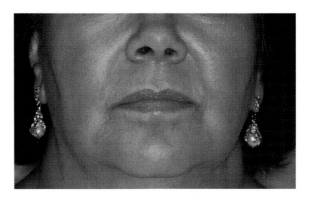

Figure 5-28

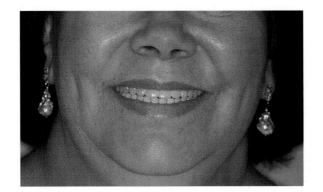

Figure 5-29

Implant-Supported Single-Tooth Prosthetics

Traditional methods of replacing individually missing teeth include removable partial dentures, tooth-supported fixed partial dentures, and resin-bonded prosthetics, such as the Maryland Bridge. The removable partial denture requires a large casting, which covers part of the palate. Clasping units may compromise esthetics, trap food, and require occasional maintenance. The stigma of having a removable prosthesis may have negative psychological effects as well. Traditional fixed prosthetics requires preparation of abutment teeth, which may have small or no restorations present. Excellent long-term function and esthetics are possible with traditional fixed prosthetics, but decay may require several total prosthetic remakes. The resin-retained prosthesis requires conservative tooth reduction but has cosmetic limitations because of metalwork that causes a graying effect on abutment teeth.

The single-tooth implant prosthesis eliminates the drawbacks inherent in a removable partial denture or in resin-bonded prosthetics. Virgin and minimally restored natural teeth are not reduced for abutments, and decay is not a factor. The single-tooth implant prosthesis is retrievable for repair or modification and may be the most cost-effective replacement over time. Drawbacks include the initial cost of surgical and prosthetic procedures. If the tooth to be replaced is still present, a 2- to 3-month healing time may be necessary after the extraction and before placing the implant. Another 4- to 6- month integration time is necessary before abutment surgery and prosthetic procedures may begin. A treatment partial, or other provisional restoration, must be used in the interim.

Several abutments and techniques are available for single-tooth restorations.

Indications for single-tooth implant-retained prosthesis include tooth loss caused by traumatically avulsed teeth, partial anodontia, cleft palate, and internal or external resorption.

Traumatically avulsed teeth may be repositioned after endodontic treatment and may be crowned if discoloration occurs. Long-term prognosis is unpredictable, and an implant prosthesis provides long-term predictability. Patients with congenitally missing teeth and unrestored remaining natural dentition are often ideal candidates for an implant prosthesis. Missing maxillary lateral incisors are found in a small percentage of the population and have often been treated by orthodontically moving cuspids into the lateral incisor position—a solution that effects an esthetic and functional compromise. Orthodontic positioning that is used to provide coronal and apical space for implant placement must be precise. Excellent esthetic results can be achieved with a final implant-retained prosthesis that restores the lateral incisor to its proper size and contour. Cleft palate patients often are missing a lateral incisor. Bone grafting, implant placement, and prosthetic single-tooth replacement can affect restoration for patients with excellent esthetics.

TREATMENT PLANNING

Mounted study casts, radiographs, and photographs are necessary for surgical and prosthetic planning. Inadequate space for implant placement may require orthodontic consultation as well. Bone quality and quantity, condition and spacing of adjacent natural dentition, intermaxillary space, and soft-tissue contours are evaluated. The surgeon evaluates space and bone quality for implant placement. Adjacent natural dentition must be caries free, with no periapical pathology. Intermaxillary space may be less than prosthetic component requirements. Orthodontics may be necessary to create adequate intermaxillary space, especially in patients with congenital anodontia. Soft-tissue deficits caused by trauma or extraction may require soft-tissue management to create ideal gingival contours. Treatment partials provide information on contours and space for the final implant-retained prosthesis and may be used as a guide for implant placement.

After surgical, orthodontic, and restorative consultations have occurred, fixture placement is completed. Seven to ten days after surgery, the treatment partial, if present, is relined with a tissue treatment material. A definitive reline is completed after healing is complete.

After adequate time for osseointegration has passed, the abutment surgery is completed. A temporary healing abutment is placed by the surgeon at this time.

CLINICAL PROCEDURES

Seven to ten days after abutment surgery an initial alginate impression is made. The treatment partial is tissue treated at this time. Soft tissues may be swollen, so abutment selection is not made until 2 weeks of additional healing have occurred.

ABUTMENT DESIGN

Single-tooth abutments must be antirotational in design. The implant-abutment interface must interlock to prevent rotation. The abutment screw must withstand high enough torquing forces to prevent it from becoming loose, yet the force must not be so strong that it will fracture the abutment screw. The Branemark CeraOne abutment was designed with those requirements in mind. It is machined with a 1 to 5 mm collar height to allow subgingival margin placement (Figs. 6-1 and 6-2). The abutment has an internal and external hexagonal design that is retained with a gold alloy screw. This design enables the abutment and implant to interlock internally, while the external hexagon keeps the implant prosthesis from rotating on the abutment. The gold alloy screw secures the implant-abutment unit and is torqued to 32 Ncm. A counter-torque instrument must be used to prevent torque transfer to the implant, which might strip the implant from the bone. Electric and manual torque drivers are available for reaching 32 Ncm. The screw is designed with a square recess that resists stripping with the high torquing forces. The previous titanium screws could only be tightened to 20 Ncm, and abutment loosening was a problem.

ABUTMENT SELECTION

Approximately 4 weeks after abutment surgery, tissue healing should be completed, and the abutment collar size is determined. The temporary healing abutment is removed using a slotted or hexagonal screwdriver. Topical anesthetic is introduced using cotton pellets that are the diameter of the abutment. The pellets prevent tissue collapse until the measurement for collar height can be determined. A periodontal probe is used to measure the distance between the fixture and the gingival surface. If the height of the healing abutment is known, the depth to the implant head can be determined by subtracting the amount of abutment above tissue from the overall abutment length. The surgeon should provide this information to the restorative dentist. After this measurement is recorded, an abutment is selected that has a collar length that is 2 to 3 mm less than the distance between the implant and the gingival surface. The screw is placed in the abutment, and the components are seated on the implant using the manual counter-torque device (Figs. 6-3 and 6-4). The square-headed screwdriver is used to tighten the gold screw (Fig. 6-5). The abutment must seat completely on the hexagonal portion of the implant. As the manual counter-torque device is rotated slightly, the abutment can be felt to slip onto the hexagonal portion of the implant. The gold alloy screw is hand tightened, and a radiograph is made, aiming the beam parallel to the implant-abutment interface to verify the seating (Figs. 6-6 and 6-7). While the radiograph is being developed, the blue nylon impression coping is placed on the external hexagonal portion of the abutment to prevent soft-tissue collapse.

The nylon impression piece is internally hexagonal to allow a press fit on the hexagonal portion of the abutment (Fig. 6-8). After radiographic verification of the abutment seating, an open window custom tray is tried in the patient's mouth to ensure the path of insertion (Fig. 6-9). Any interferences with the tray placement are eliminated. A medium viscosity vinyl polysiloxane impression material is used to make the impression (Fig. 6-10). After the appropriate adhesive is applied on the tray, the impression material is loaded into the tray; it is also distributed around the impression coping using a syringe. Hydrostatic pressure and tissue pressure may slightly unseat the coping; therefore the coping is reseated before placing the impression tray in the patient's mouth. The tray is seated, engaging the impression coping through the tray window. Finger pressure should be maintained on the impression coping until the impression material has set. Excess impression material is removed from around the coping, and autopolymerizing resin is used to secure the coping to the impression tray (Fig. 6-11). After the impression has set, it is removed from the mouth (Fig. 6-12). An interocclusal record, a shade selection, and an impression of the opposing arch are made at this time. A temporary crown or the healing abutment is replaced.

POURING THE MASTER CAST

The implant replica is placed on the inferior surface of the CeraOne impression coping (Figs. 6-13 and 6-14), engaging

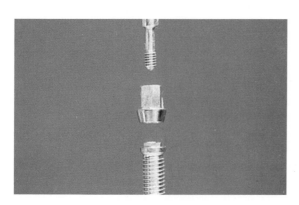

Figure 6-1

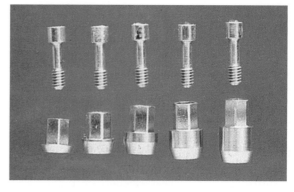

Figure 6-2

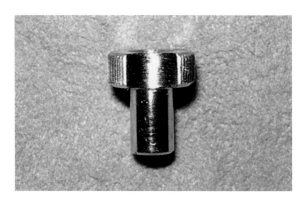

Figure 6-3

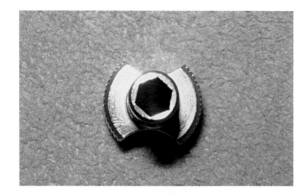

Figure 6-4

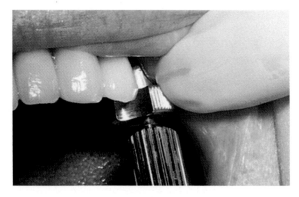

Figure 6-5

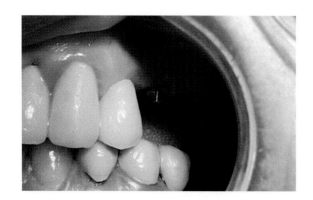

Figure 6-6

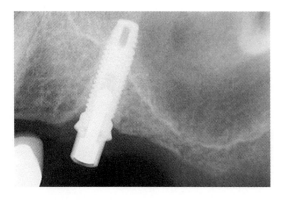

Figure 6-7

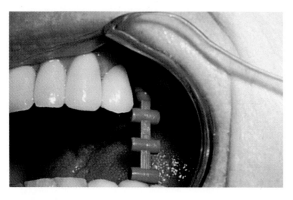

Figure 6-8

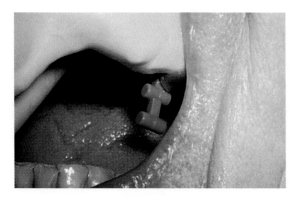

Figure 6-9

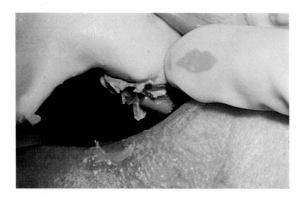

Figure 6-10

the internal hex, and it is held in place by a compression fit of the impression coping. The cast can be poured by using either of the following two methods:

1. Before the master cast is poured, a soft-tissue conditioning material can be painted at the gingival area to create a flexible zone around the abutment analog (Fig. 6-15).
2. A thin layer of utility wax is placed on the gingival area of the impression coping to inhibit the coping from adhering to the diestone of the cast (Figs. 6-16 and 6-17). This eliminates the possibility of fracturing the master cast upon separation of the impression tray from the cast.

If the second method is used, a special treatment of the master cast is performed to allow visualization of the interface between the abutment analog and the prosthesis. Diestone is removed from the lingual surface of the implant replica site. The master cast is mounted on a semiadjustable articulator.

OTHER LABORATORY PROCEDURES

Ceramic caps made from densely sintered aluminum oxide are specially designed for use with the CeraOne abutments (Figs. 6-18 and 6-19). This all-ceramic core material offers both optimal esthetics and strength. The cap is available in a

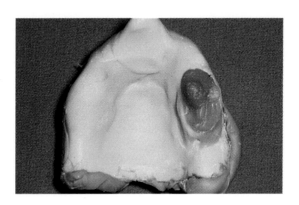

Figure 6-11

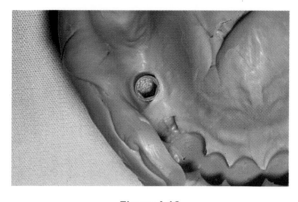

Figure 6-12

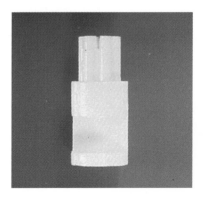

Figure 6-13

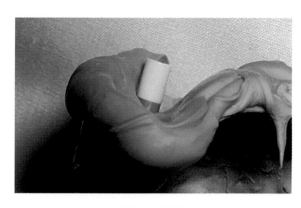

Figure 6-14

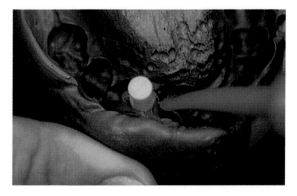

Figure 6-15

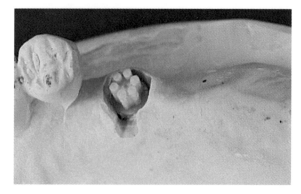

Figure 6-16

short and a long length; the selected cap should ensure as much support as possible for the finished crown while it allows for an even layer of porcelain (Figs. 6-20 and 6-21).

The core is manufactured in one shade and can be adjusted by adding an aluminum oxide-core porcelain, such as Vita Dur N HiCeram core material, which is reinforced with 45% to 50% aluminum oxide particles. The porcelain must be well condensed and vacuum fired to eliminate pores in the crystalline ceramic (Fig. 6-22). An all-ceramic crown porcelain, such as Vita Dur N, must be used and can be directly stacked to the core material. The porcelain should be manipulated while wet and not allowed to dry out. Firing should be done slowly to allow any porosities to disappear. The porcelain must not reach the maximum firing temperature before 5 minutes has elapsed. Prolonged firing under vacuum at the maximum firing temperature should be avoided, since the glass phase can form bubbles or swell at these temperatures.

To avoid porcelain with pores, the vacuum must be broken when the aluminum oxide-reinforced porcelain reaches the firing temperature recommended by the manufacturer. After the vacuum has been broken, the aluminum oxide-reinforced porcelain can be safely fired at atmospheric pressure for a long time. If the firing times are too short, the glass phase does not have time to become viscous enough to flow and bond

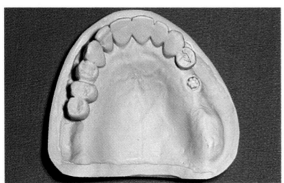

Figure 6-17

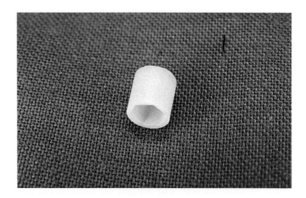

Figure 6-18

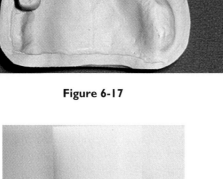

Figure 6-19

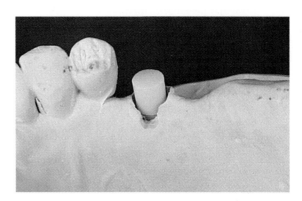

Figure 6-20

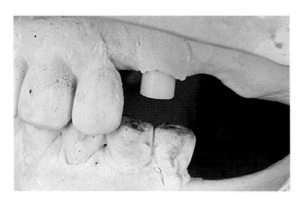

Figure 6-21

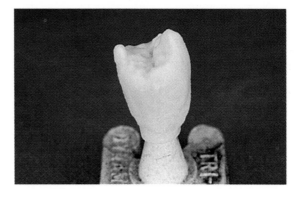

Figure 6-22

chemically to the aluminum oxide crystals. Tests have shown that complete bonding to the cap can be achieved after 2 minutes.

The cores are adjusted (if necessary) with a diamond bur. The porcelain will bond chemically to the core, so the surface need not be ground to obtain an even porcelain application. The thickness of the core wall should not be less than 0.5 mm on the larger surfaces. For small areas, the cap wall thickness can be slightly less. Before firing takes place, the core should be washed in a solution of diluted hydrofluoric acid for 5 minutes and then carefully cleaned in an ultrasonic bath. As an alternative the core can also be cleaned by blasting with pure aluminum oxide powder.

Core material is applied in two firings. The porcelain powder should be mixed with the liquid supplied by the manufacturer. The first layer of porcelain powder should be thin. A smooth contour is developed while wetting the entire surface to prevent porosity. The porcelain should be fired at 1130° C. The second layer of porcelain is fired at 1120° C, and after this firing the surface should be similar to an eggshell to spread reflected light better.

When the dentin material is fired, work is facilitated by applying a little petroleum jelly to the replica to help keep the crown in place and to minimize the risk of the porcelain attaching itself to the inside of the crown. The firing is done carefully so that the jelly will not get on the outside of the ceramic core. The crown is built up using the traditional porcelain-layering techniques. The crown is glazed after clinical trial fitting has been performed (Figs. 6-23 and 6-24).

BISQUE TRIAL FITTING AND DELIVERY

The finished prosthesis is first seated on an extra CeraOne abutment to evaluate the fit. Retention and complete seating are evaluated. Internal debris or flashing may prevent complete seating on the abutment. A disclosing solution is used to show the areas of interference, and these are removed. The healing cap or provisional restoration is removed. If not previously completed on bisque evaluation, the prosthesis is seated, the proximal contacts are checked and adjusted, and a radiograph is made to survey the complete seating. The

occlusion is then adjusted to allow light contact; however, no contact is allowed in eccentric positions. After the restoration is reglazed and polished (if necessary) it is ready for cementation. When the restoration is porcelain fused to metal, a lingual vent hole is cut through the metal approximately 1 1/2 mm in diameter. This allows an escape for excess cement while providing a purchase point for tapping the restoration off if necessary. Properly done, this will retain the retrievability of the restoration if complications occur. Excess cement may be impossible to access subgingivally, and soft tissue infections are common when subgingival cement is present. A non-retrievable prosthesis in this situation will require surgically accessing the interface to remove cement. A retrievable restoration eliminates this problem. The electric torque converter with the square-headed driver is used for final tightening of the gold alloy screw (Figs. 6-25 and 6-26). The counter-torque device must be used to prevent stripping the fixture from the bone. The counter-torque device is first seated on the abutment and checked for lack of rotation. The square-headed driver is used to engage the gold alloy screw (Fig. 6-27). The electric torque converter is set to 32 Ncm at the low setting. The foot pedal is then used to completely tighten the screw. A cotton pellet is placed over the gold screw inside the abutment. The choice of cement depends on retention between the abutment and the prosthesis. In many instances, temporary cement will retain the restoration and allow for possible retrieval of the unit if necessary. If retention is not high, a more permanent cement must be used. Only a thin layer of cement is used inside the restoration to prevent subgingival cement, which may be difficult to remove. After cementation, hygiene instructions are given to the patient. The single-tooth prosthesis is checked according to protocol at follow-up appointments (Figs. 6-28 and 6-29).

CERAONE METAL COPING
Waxing Procedure

When the CeraOne is waxed with a metal coping, the design and fabrication of the substructure must be considered. A plastic burnout replica pattern is available for casting a CeraOne metal coping.

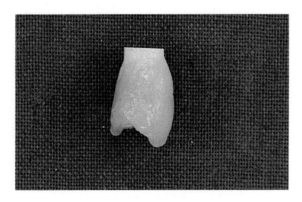

Figure 6-23

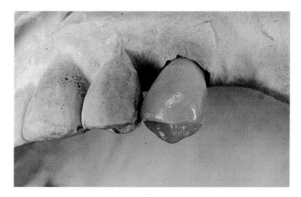

Figure 6-24

The burnout replica pattern is placed on the plastic abutment replica, and the pattern is adjusted for the metal and porcelain additions. The burnout replica is shortened to allow adequate porcelain thickness. The area around the abutment replica and burnout replica is lubricated on the master cast to facilitate easy removal. Inlay wax is applied to the burnout replica, and a full contour waxing is completed. The tissue emergence profiles are established. The wax pattern is cut back for proper thickness of porcelain application (Figs. 6-30 and 6-31). The facial ceramic metal junction can be carried subgingivally to allow development of the emergence profile (Fig. 6-32). The wax pattern is indirectly sprued (Fig. 6-33)

with an 8-gauge sprue at the lingual surface and removed from the plastic abutment replica.

Phosphate investment with proper expansion is recommended to ensure a precise fit between the fabricated casting and the CeraOne abutment replica. A manufacturer's investment procedure is recommended. An alloy is selected with the tensile strength of around 150,000 Ncm. (Alloys designed for ceramic application have a greater tensile strength, thus their selection when porcelain is to be applied is recommended.) An extra CeraOne abutment should be used to verify fit and interface during the reclaiming and metal finishing of the cast coping. Interferences to smooth seating are

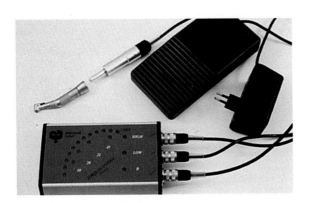

Figure 6-25

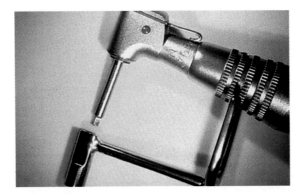

Figure 6-26

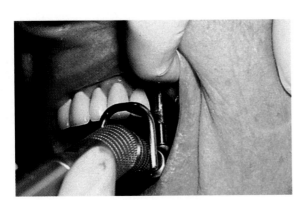

Figure 6-27

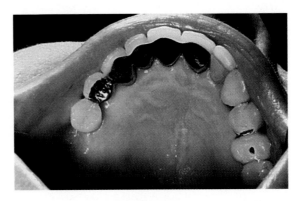

Figure 6-28

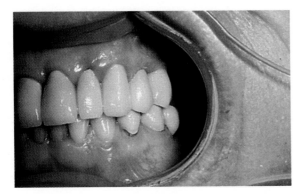

Figure 6-29

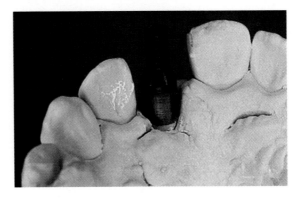

Figure 6-30

identified under magnification and eliminated. No metal try-in is needed because it is a single unit, so standard procedures for porcelain application are completed (Figs. 6-34 and 6-35).

CLINICAL DELIVERY

Clinical procedures for the CeraOne metal coping have been discussed previously (the ceramic cap procedure). Occlusion is adjusted to allow light centric occlusion contact with no contact in any excursive movements. Radiographic verification should be performed to ensure that the casting is seated onto the abutment and that the interface between the cast coping and the abutment is closed. If the occlusion requires

adjustment, it is accomplished after verification of seating. The completed restoration is shown in Fig. 6-36.

A metal-supported ceramic prosthesis is recommended for all posterior single-tooth restorations. Figs. 6-37 to 6-39 demonstrate ceramic metal prosthesis for congenital anodontia. Figs. 6-40 to 6-45 show single molar replacement in the maxillary posterior. The patient in Figs. 6-46 to 6-52 had a bone graft to repair a cleft palate defect. After the grafting procedure, implant placement and single-tooth replacement was done. Figs. 6-53 to 6-62 illustrate fabrication and replacement of tooth #6, using a machined gold cylinder rather than the plastic burnout pattern or ceramic cap. Conventional

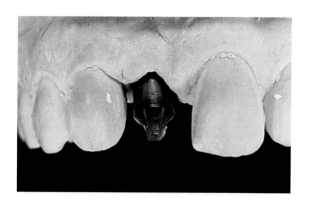

Figure 6-31

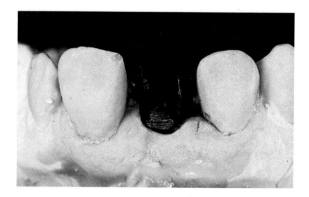

Figure 6-32

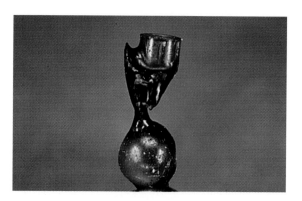

Figure 6-33

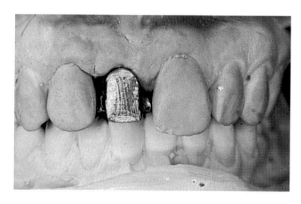

Figure 6-34

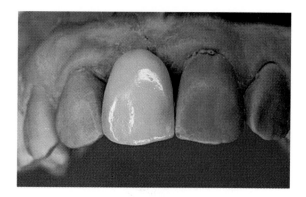

Figure 6-35

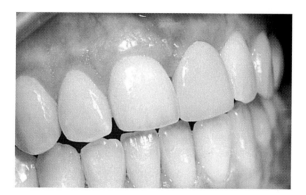

Figure 6-36

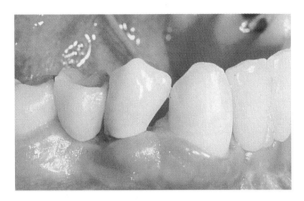

Figure 6-37

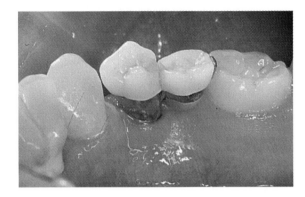

Figure 6-38

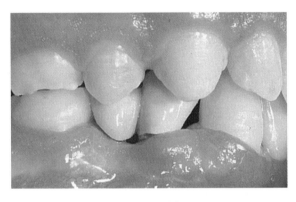

Figure 6-39

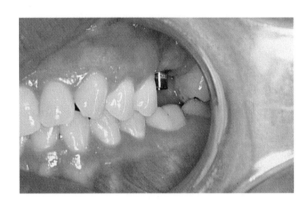

Figure 6-40

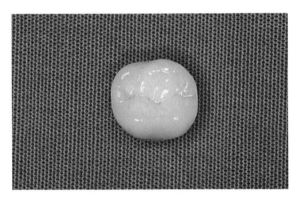

Figure 6-41

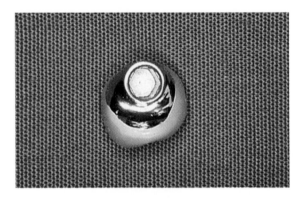

Figure 6-42

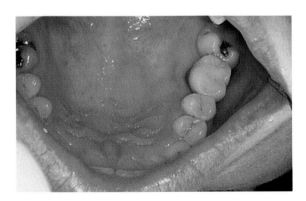

Figure 6-43

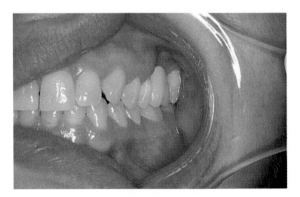

Figure 6-44

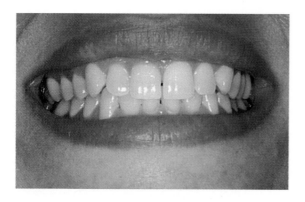

Figure 6-45

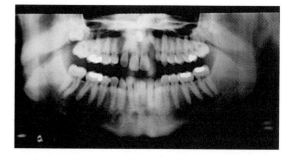

Figure 6-46

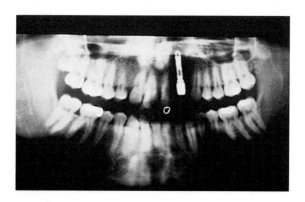

Figure 6-47

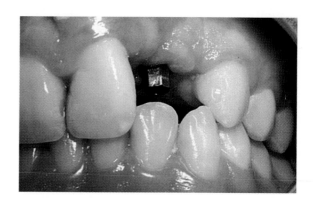

Figure 6-48

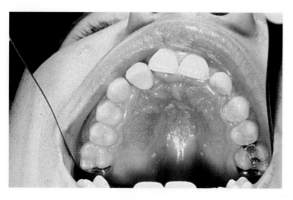

Figure 6-49

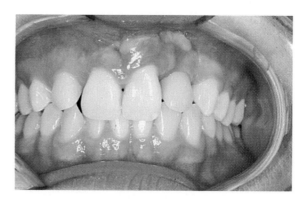

Figure 6-50

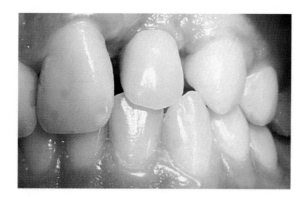

Figure 6-51

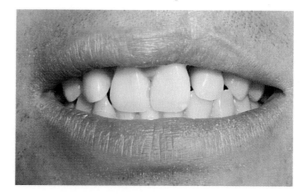

Figure 6-52

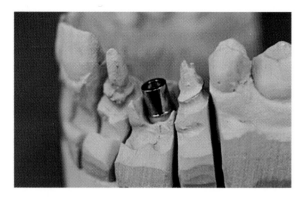

Figure 6-53

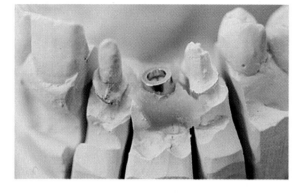

Figure 6-54

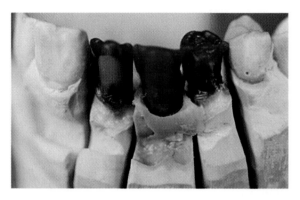

Figure 6-55

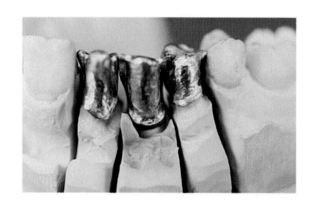

Figure 6-56

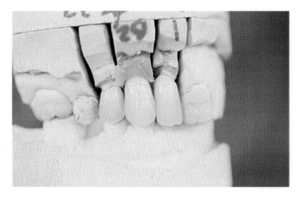

Figure 6-57

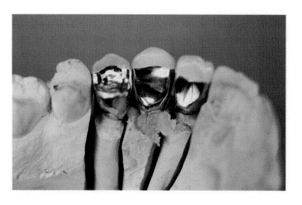

Figure 6-58

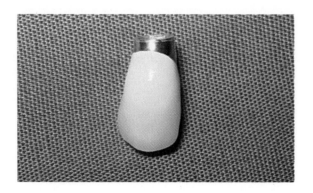

Figure 6-59

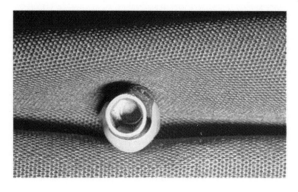

Figure 6-60

porcelain-to-metal restorations on teeth #5 and #7 were completed as well.

SOFT-TISSUE MANAGEMENT

Restoring the maxillary anterior teeth when a high smile line exists requires special procedures to create natural esthetics. The level, curvature, and contour of the gingival margin of the prosthetic tooth must match the contralateral tooth and blend with adjacent gingival contours. The surgeon should leave excess tissue for expansion with the provisional restoration (Fig. 6-63). The implant position, as seen on the working cast (Fig. 6-64), is slightly palatal. Provisional restora-

tions are made on the working cast. Methylmethacrylate resin is added to the gingival buccal portion of the provisional, which when seated will cause the tissues to move buccally and gingivally while initially blanching (Figs. 6-65 and 6-66). The provisional is modified weekly until the gingival buccal contour of the tissue blends with the adjacent dentition. Removal of the provisionals shows how tissue has been expanded (Fig. 6-67). An impression of the provisional is then made and used by the laboratory technician as a guide for making the definitive restoration (Fig. 6-68). The contour, level, and curvature of the gingiva blends with the adjacent teeth after seating of the definitive prosthesis (Figs. 6-69 and 6-70).

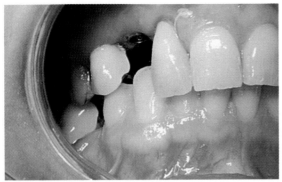

Figure 6-61

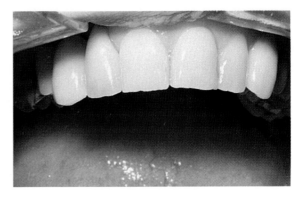

Figure 6-62

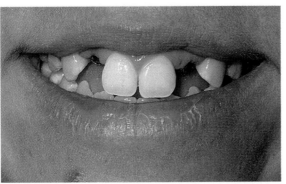

Figure 6-63

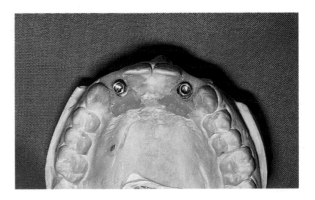

Figure 6-64

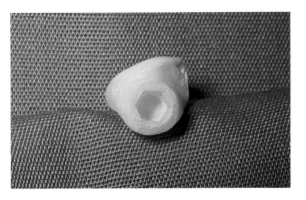

Figure 6-65

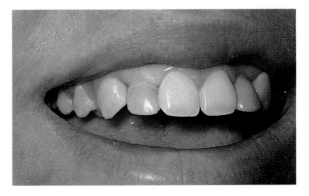

Figure 6-66

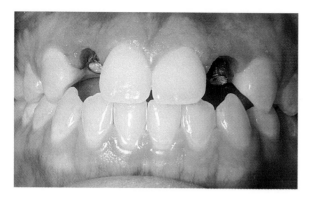

Figure 6-67

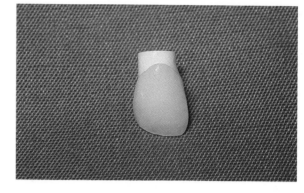

Figure 6-68

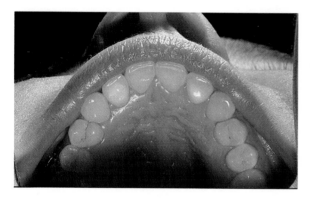

Figure 6-69

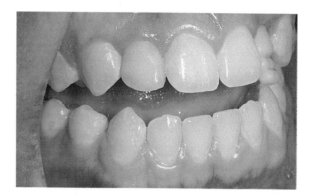

Figure 6-70

Chapter 7

CerAdapt Abutment

Abraham Ingber
Vincent Prestipino
Joseph Kravitz

Osseointegrated dental implants continue to demonstrate success for both partially and fully edentulous patients. However, it is difficult to achieve predictable long-term esthetic results in the esthetic zone because of soft- and hard-tissue deformities and technique-sensitive clinical and laboratory procedures. The benefit of an implant option in this zone is often ignored by the dentist because of the perceived risks of these procedures and intimidation from complex component parts with minimum esthetic features. Proper diagnosis and treatment planning of the future implant site requires an understanding of the following parameters: lip posture, gingival health and architecture, hard- and soft-tissue volume, and implant position. The use of the CerAdapt abutment will improve esthetics of the implant restoration in some clinical situations.

The CerAdapt abutment was developed[1] to simplify the implant restorative procedures (Fig. 7-1). This abutment system is part of the Simpler in Practice treatment concept (recently introduced by Nobel Biocare), which uses traditional crown and bridge procedures to manage the implant restoration. The abutment was designed to be highly esthetic and versatile to allow the dentist to achieve a predictable cosmetic result with a high degree of confidence. This is accomplished with a tooth-colored, precision-milled, single ceramic component, which can be prepared, customized, and adapted to variations in implant position as well as peri-implant soft-tissue anatomy.

SOFT- AND HARD-TISSUE ESTHETIC CONSIDERATIONS

Patients demand and expect esthetic results from fixed and removable partial dentures as well as implant-supported restorations. A compelling smile is illuminating and pleasing when there is no distraction from compromised health, harmony, balance, color, shape, and size in the perioral ambience. An evaluation of the smile line and lip posture can help determine the esthetic risks for the patient and the dentist. It is important to inform patients of these risks, to discuss unrealistic expectations, and to gain consent. A patient with a high lip line is obviously more difficult to treat, requires a commitment to the esthetic criteria, and demands the most from the surgeon, restorative dentist, and technician (Fig.

7-2). A patient with a low lip line can be easier to manage but does not preclude an esthetic outcome.

It is known that healthy tissue with optimum architecture around dental implants is necessary for a successful esthetic result. Implant surgery may affect the surrounding soft- and hard-tissue architecture adversely. It is helpful to understand the characteristics and biology of the soft and hard tissues and their reaction to surgical insults before therapy. Proper analysis of the soft-tissue type and evaluation of the implant site with radiographs and study casts can reduce these untoward effects.[2]

There are two types of periodontal tissues: thick flat and thin scalloped[3] (Fig. 7-3, *A* and *B*). The thick flat type of periodontium is dense and fibrotic with large amounts of masticatory mucosa, characterized by square crown forms and large contact areas. This tissue type is preferred and responds to surgical injury and insults by the formation of infra-bony pockets and hyperplastic tissue. Generally the healing response is uneventful. In contrast, the thin scalloped tissue type is delicate and friable with small amounts of masticatory mucosa. This tissue type is more difficult to manage and reacts to insults with facial and interproximal recession.

Ridge deformities and extraction-site defects present a challenge to the final implant restoration.[4] There are many successful surgical augmentation procedures that are available (e.g., guided bone regeneration, guided tissue regeneration, and subepithelial connective tissue grafts) (Fig. 7-4, *A* to *C*). However, these surgical augmentation results can be less then ideal and at times unpredictable. Therapeutic goals should include optimum preprosthetic conditions. These conditions are guaranteed by site development before implant placement and the "15% volume rule." This recommendation to the surgeon to overbuild the recipient site by approximately 15% in volume will counteract the postoperative graft resorption and create a more favorable site for implant placement and ideal crown construction (Fig. 7-5).

IMPLANT POSITIONING

Ideal implant position is key to the success of the final restoration. This can be accomplished through proper planning from both restorative and surgical points of view. The use of a diagnostic wax-up and surgical template with implant positioning guides or direction indicators is critical (Fig. 7-6).

The template should be a duplicate of the final crown form and offer the surgeon good visualization and a three-dimensional orientation to the surgical site for the starting point and twist drill preparation (see Fig. 7-5). The implant position in the anterior zone should be placed approximately 2 to 4 mm below the ideal gingival margin so that there is sufficient room to allow for transition of the prepared ceramic abutment from a circular implant to a natural emergence contour (Fig. 7-7). The body of the implant should be placed as far labial as possible so the ceramic abutment can be prepared with flat labial emergence to prevent excessive crown contours, shadows, and hygiene problems (Fig. 7-8). The implant

should also be directed toward the incisal or lingual incisal edge for cement-retained restorations. This orientation maintains sufficient thickness of the prepared ceramic abutment at the gingival margin for optimum strength and for ideal contours of the final cemented restoration (Fig. 7-9, *A* and *B*).

CERADAPT ABUTMENT
Composition

The CerAdapt abutment system was developed[5] to simplify the most challenging esthetic implant restorations[6] (Fig. 7-10). The abutment is an all-ceramic alternative to metal abutments. The CerAdapt abutment is a premachined,

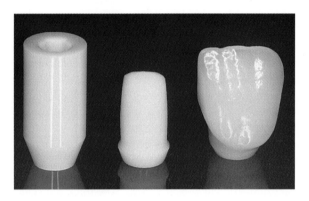

Figure 7-1

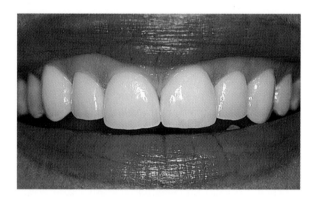

Figure 7-2

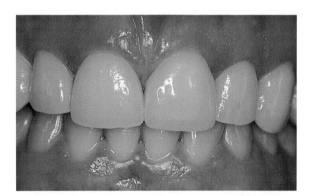

Figure 7-3, A

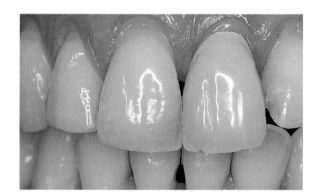

Figure 7-3, B

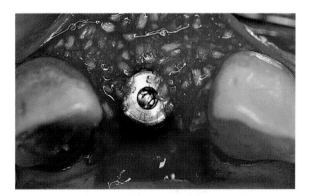

Figure 7-4, A

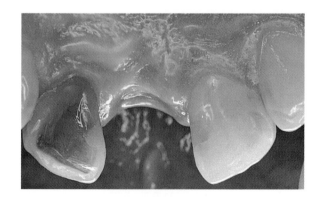

Figure 7-4, B

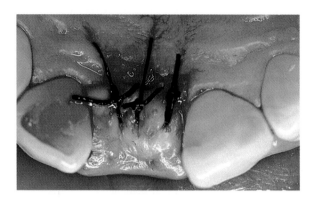

Figure 7-4, C

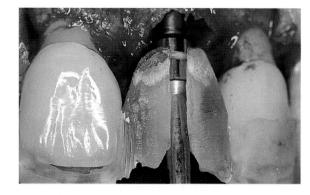

Figure 7-5

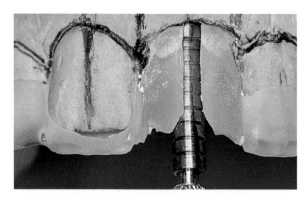

Figure 7-6

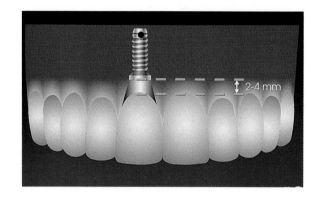

Figure 7-7

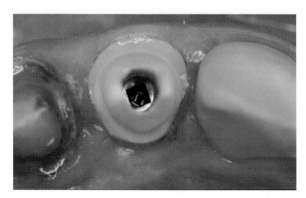

Figure 7-8

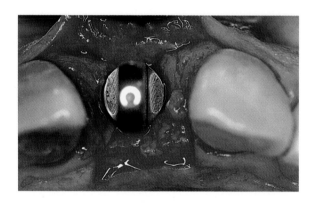

Figure 7-9, A

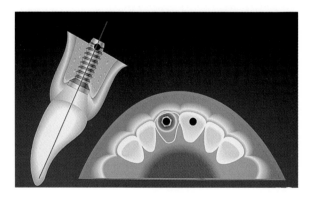

Figure 7-9, B

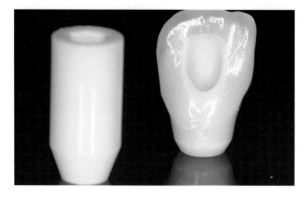

Figure 7-10

precision-milled abutment made to fit the implant hex. It is made of densely sintered 99.8% pure aluminum oxide. Particles of aluminum oxide are pressed into the desired shape and subjected to sintering temperatures of 2050° C. During sintering, the aluminum oxide shrinks, resulting in a pore-free, strong, wear-resistant, stable bioceramic material (Fig. 7-11). Andersson and Oden show flexural strengths of 690 MPa and demonstrate that the abutment can withstand tremendous loads without fracturing.[7]

This abutment is nonmetallic, noncorrosive, and biocompatible, and it develops a mucosa barrier similar to that of titanium abutments. The soft-tissue response is excellent (Fig. 7-12, A). The CerAdapt abutment has unique optical qualities. It is tooth colored and has light-diffusion properties through the abutment and through the surrounding tissue. These benefits offer several advantages over similar metallic abutments and clearly make it easier to achieve a more natural and esthetic implant crown (Fig. 7-12, B).

The CerAdapt abutment can be used for implant-supported single- and multiple-tooth restorations in the anterior, canine, and premolar regions on Branemark System implants, regular platform. The abutments can be prepared into the desired shape by the dental technician and refined intraorally by the dentist for cemented restorations, or porcelain can be directly applied to the abutment for a screw-retained restoration (Fig. 7-13). These options and the custom design capability of the abutment allow for a great deal of flexibility and adaptability in shape and color, thereby facilitating an optimum esthetic result.

SEQUENCED CLINICAL AND LABORATORY PROCEDURES
Restorative Procedures

The proper pretreatment evaluation of the implant patient is critical for a successful result. The surgeon (the one who places the implant), restorative dentist, and dental technician should develop a comprehensive treatment plan that clearly identifies the responsibilities of each member of the treatment team.

The restorative dentist makes maxillary and mandibular preliminary full-arch impressions, develops diagnostic casts, and selects the proper shade. The diagnostic casts are sent to the laboratory for full wax-up and the fabrication of a clear surgical template. The template should be a duplicate of the final crown form and offer the surgeon good visualization and three-dimensional orientation to the surgical site for starting point and twist-drill preparation (see Fig. 7-6). The surgical template is sent to the surgeon.

Surgical Procedures

The surgeon installs the implant using the surgical template. Just before placement of the cover screw, a implant level reg-

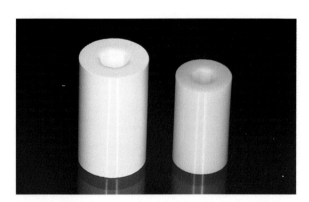

Figure 7-11

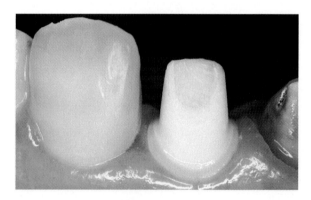

Figure 7-12, A

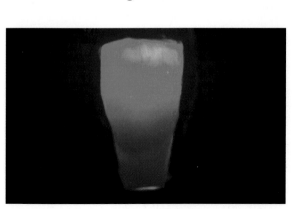

Figure 7-12, B

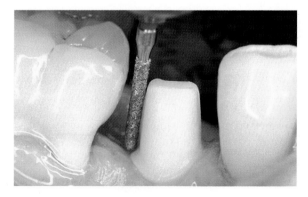

Figure 7-13

istration is made using a plastic implant registration coping (Nobel Biocare SDCA838). Fixture registration copings are available for all implant sizes: narrow platform (NP), regular platform (RP), and wide platform (WP) (Fig. 7-14, *A* and *B*). A screw-retained titanium implant registration coping (Nobel Biocare DCA1040) is also available.

The implant registration coping is carefully rotated to align the coping hex with the implant hex. The coping is pressed and snapped into place, ensuring that the coping is completely seated. The surgeon, using an auto-mix syringe, dispenses a viscous vinyl polysiloxane silicone impression material (Blu-Mousse Super-Fast, by Parkell, Framingdale, N.J.) onto the occlusal two-thirds of the registration coping and the occlusal surfaces of the adjacent two teeth. This material sets in 30 seconds and registers the proper relation of the implant to the teeth (Fig. 7-15, *A* to *C*). This registration index is easily retrieved by pulling on the plastic coping and setting it aside for delivery to the dental technician. The technician is informed which platform was used (narrow, regular, or wide). The cover screw is placed on the implant, and the flap is closed.

Laboratory Procedures

The dental technician retrieves the disinfected implant registration coping/silicone assembly and carefully attaches an implant replica of the appropriate platform, making sure that the implant replica is fully seated (Fig. 7-16, *A* and *B*). The diagnostic cast previously used for fabrication of the surgical guide is prepared. Using a laboratory carbide drill, a socket is prepared into the stone cast for the registration coping/implant replica assembly. The assembly is placed into the prepared socket to check for any possible interferences. The socket is adequate when the registration coping/implant replica silicone assembly can be fully seated on the stone cast teeth without interference from the socket borders and the implant replica. An access window for luting resin is prepared on the cast apical and lingual to the implant replica position. With the assembly fully seated, acrylic resin is applied into the window to lute the replica to the stone cast.

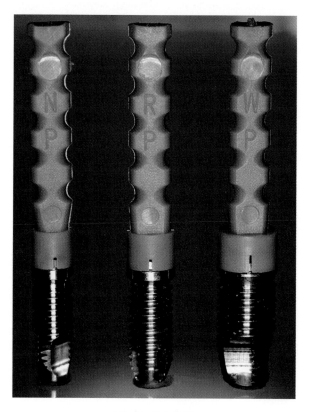

Figure 7-14, A

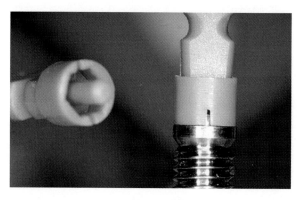

Figure 7-14, B

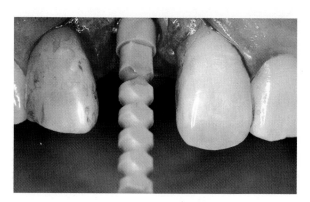

Figure 7-15, A

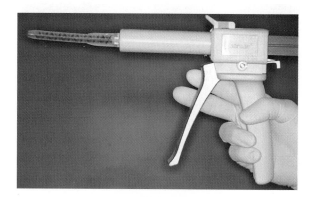

Figure 7-15, B

When the acrylic is set, the registration coping assembly is removed. The master cast is complete with proper replication of the implant position (Fig. 7-17, *A* to *E*).

Abutment Preparation Design

The technician selects the CerAdapt abutment and attempts to connect it to the replica on the stone cast with a titanium laboratory screw (Fig. 7-18). As the abutment is seated, interferences are noted and the abutment is prepared and relieved until it is fully seated onto the replica (Fig. 7-19). The CerAdapt is prepared with a high-speed handpiece under copious water irrigation. The abutment is reduced to the desired height and shaped with coarse-grit diamond burs. Diamond wheels are used for overall fast reduction, and tapered diamonds with rounded or chamfer tips are used for axial wall preparation (Fig. 7-20). Minimum abutment dimensional requirements are identified in the illustrations (Fig. 7-21). The preparation should leave a minimum of 7 mm abutment height on one side. The diameter should not be less than 4 mm with a minimum sidewall thickness of 0.7 mm. The abutment should not be angled more then 30 degrees from the long axis of the implant.

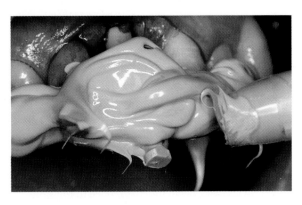

Figure 7-15, C

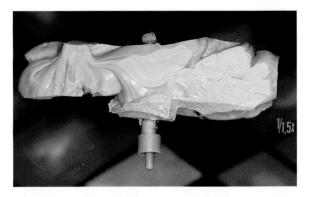

Figure 7-16, A

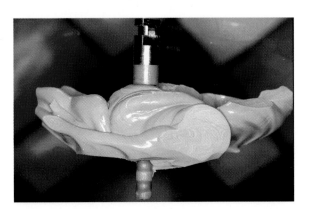

Figure 7-16, B

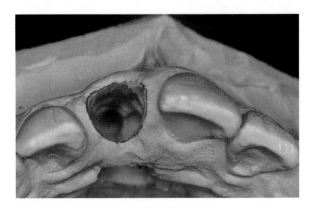

Figure 7-17, A

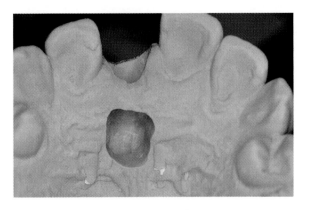

Figure 7-17, B

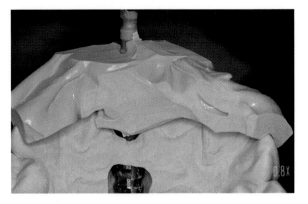

Figure 7-17, C

The reduction and shape of the abutment depend on the style of the final crown. In the case of the screw-retained crown, aluminous porcelain (Procera All Ceram) is stacked directly onto the prepared abutment and shaped into the final crown form and then stained, glazed, and finished. The final screw-retained crown is sent to the surgeon (Fig. 7-22, *A* and *B*).

In the case of the cement over crowns, the abutment is prepared and reduced into the desired root-tooth-prepped shape and is stained, glazed, and finished (Fig. 7-23, *A*). If after abutment preparation the emerging cervical contours are incomplete or inadequate to support the cement over the crown, then aluminous porcelain (Procera All Ceram) can be stacked and fired into the desired root shape, then stained, glazed, and finished (Fig. 7-23, *B*). When the abutment is completed, a provisional restoration is fabricated. The provisional restoration and the custom-prepped ceramic abutment are sent to the surgeon (Fig. 7-23, *C*).

Surgical Procedures

The surgeon performs the uncovery procedure, making sure that the implant is free of any soft tissue or bone fragments.

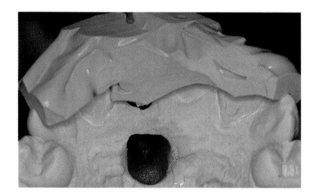

Figure 7-17, D

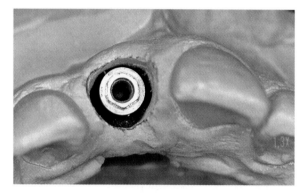

Figure 7-17, E

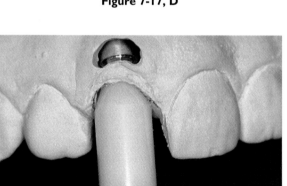

Figure 7-18

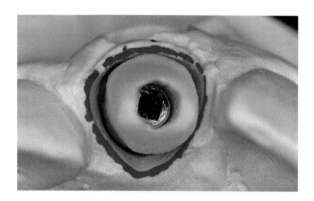

Figure 7-19

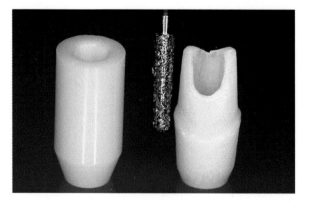

Figure 7-20

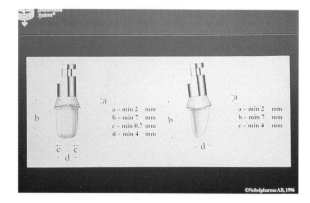

Figure 7-21

The sterilized final screw-retained crown or the custom abutment with the provisional restoration and the gold abutment screw is delivered to the implant using a hand-held screwdriver (Fig. 7-24, *A* and *B*). The gold screw is hand torqued until the initial resistance is noted. A radiograph is taken to verify complete seating of the abutment. At this point, if the abutment-tissue relationship is correct, the surgeon may use the counter-torque device and electric torque controller to deliver the proper torque value. However, in most cases, the peri-implant tissues are left to heal for 6 to 8 weeks, and the final adjustments are made by the restorative dentist.

Restorative Procedures

If necessary, final modifications are made to the abutment, final screw-retained crown, and/or provisional restoration. The counter-torque device must be used when the final torque value is applied to the gold alloy abutment screw. Gutta percha and composite resin are used to seal the access channel. Slight refinement of the abutment margin can be

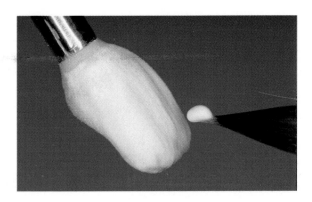

Figure 7-22, A

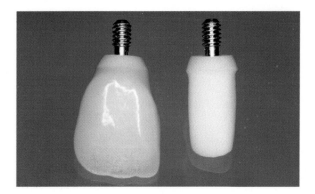

Figure 7-22, B

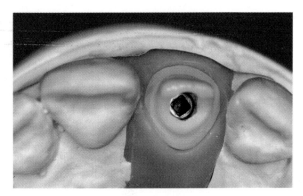

Figure 7-23, A

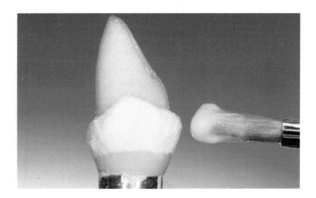

Figure 7-23, B

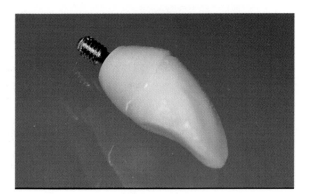

Figure 7-23, C

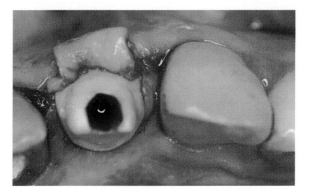

Figure 7-24, A

made, and standard procedures and techniques can be followed for the final impression and fabrication of the final restoration. For cementation of the final restoration, any conventional luting agent can be used. Temporary luting agents may be preferred for a bridge if retrievability is desired.

CERADAPT ABUTMENT CLINICAL APPLICATIONS

The CerAdapt abutment can be prepared and used in two alternative ways. The screw-retained crown is used when direct retrievability is desired and the access channel has a favorable direction. After preparation adequate for porcelain veneering, the porcelain is fired directly onto the CerAdapt abutment to form the screw-retained crown. The crown is secured to the implant with a gold alloy abutment screw (Fig. 7-25, *A* to *C*).

The cemented crown is preferred and used when the screw access channel is somewhat maligned or when a screw access hole in the crown is not desired. The CerAdapt abutment is prepared like a natural tooth and then secured to the implant. A conventional impression is made for the fabrication of the final cemented crown (Fig. 7-26, *A* to *D*).

REFERENCES

1. Ingber A, Prestipino V: New technology: high-strength ceramic abutment, *Dental Implantology Update* 2:70, 1991.
2. Jansen C, Weisgold A: Presurgical treatment planning for the anterior single-tooth implant restoration, *Compendium* 16(8):746, 1995
3. Olsson M, Lindhe J: Periodontal characteristics in individuals with varying forms of the upper central incisors, *J Clin Periodont* 18:78, 1991.
4. Salama H, Salama M: The role of orthodontic extrusive remodeling in the enhancement of soft and hard tissue profiles prior to implant placement: a systematic approach of extraction site defects, *Int J Perio Restor Dent* 13(4):312, 1993.
5. Prestipino V, Ingber A: Esthetic high-strength implant abutments: Part I, *J Esthet Dent* 5(1):29, 1993.
6. Prestipino V, Ingber A: Esthetic high-strength implant abutments: Part II, *J Esthet Dent* 5(2):63, 1993.
7. Andersson M, Oden A: A new all-ceramic crown: a dense-sintered, high purity alumina coping with porcelain, *Acta Odontol Scand* 51:59, 1993.

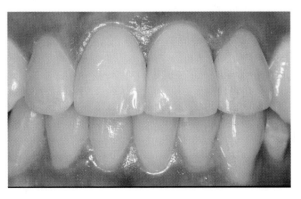

Figure 7-24, B

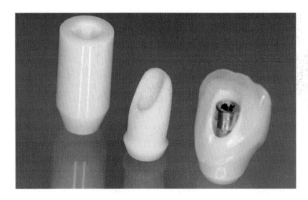

Figure 7-25, A

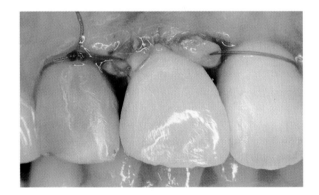

Figure 7-25, B

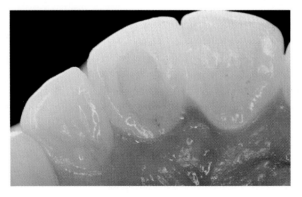

Figure 7-25, C

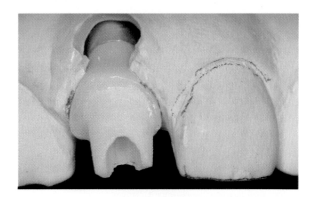

Figure 7-26, A

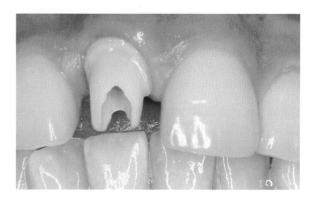

Figure 7-26, B

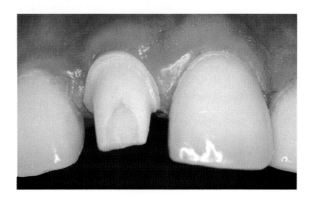

Figure 7-26, C

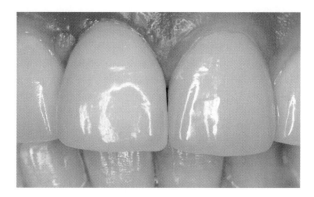

Figure 7-26, D

CHAPTER 8   Partially Edentulous Implant Prosthetics

Partial edentulism has traditionally been treated with conventional fixed prosthetics when adequate natural tooth abutments are available to support the edentulous span. Removable partial dentures provide a more economic restorative option with severe inherent disadvantages. Retentive elements may compromise esthetics, trap food, and require occasional adjustment to maintain retention. Masticatory efficiency is less than with fixed alternatives, and major connectors may never be completely accepted by patients. Psychological problems associated with removable prosthetics make this the least desirable form of tooth replacement.

Tooth-supported fixed partial dentures provide more functional and esthetic replacements for missing teeth. Abutment preparation weakens teeth and increases susceptibility to decay, and abutment teeth may require root canal therapy from the trauma of preparation. Replacement of traditional fixed prosthetics over a patient's lifetime is common and expensive.

The implant-supported fixed prosthesis has many advantages. Implant loss resulting from decay and periodontal involvement are eliminated. Retrievable designs allow prosthetic removal for repair, component replacement, and modification, greatly reducing expenses compared with traditional bridge remakes. Virgin teeth are spared preparation. These advantages make the implant prosthesis the most predictable and cost-effective prosthetic option for many patients wih missing teeth or teeth with a poor prognosis.

TREATMENT PLANNING

The number of implants needed is determined by the number and position of missing teeth; available width, height and quality of bone in the edentulous area; and the edentulous arch form. Wide diameter and wide platform implants are used where indicated for mechanical advantage. Complications with component loosening, screw fracture, and even implant fracture can occur in posterior implant prosthetics by two or three standard diameter implants placed in a straight line. Chapter 9 discusses, in depth, treatment planning using the new wide platform components. Increased screw diameter and improved alloys allow much higher torque application for resistance to component loosening.

Other parameters affecting treatment planning include intermaxillary space, height of smile line, and bony- and soft-tissue contours in the edentulous area. An intraoral examination is completed with periodontal charting, caries examination, and cancer screening. Radiographs are made, including panorex and periapical films. Mounted diagnostic casts are also needed. The patient's expectations and finances affect treatment plans as well. After surgical consultation the restorative dentist and surgeon together examine diagnostic casts and radiographs. The laboratory technician may need to be involved in treatment planning if there are any questions about prosthetic design and component choice.

Ideal anatomy should exist for implant placement. Bone and soft-tissue grafting is incorporated as part of the treatment plan. There is no reason to place implants in less than ideal position. Orthodontic discrepancy, both dental and skeletal, may need to be addressed, as well as the periodontal and endodontic prognosis of the whole mouth.

Implant manufacturers and dental laboratories will offer to provide treatment plans for patients for the inexperienced practitioner. Advertisements are seen that offer complete treatment planning services, including estimates for treatment. Each patient must be evaluated on an individual basis by surgeons and restorative dentists. Dental laboratories do not understand bone biology or surgical and prosthodontic needs of patients. If a dentist does not understand the treatment planning parameters, the case should be referred to specialists for treatment.

After the treatment plan is finalized, surgical templates are made to aid the surgeon in implant placement.

After the implants are placed, a healing time of 7 to 10 days is necessary without a prosthesis being worn. The existing definitive or treatment partial is relieved and relined with a tissue-conditioning material. This lining is replaced as needed until healing is complete. A more definitive reline is completed at this time. The patient is advised to return to the clinic for prosthesis adjustment at the first sign of soreness or irritation.

The abutment operation is completed at the proper time, followed by 7 to 10 days without prosthesis. The prosthesis is relieved, allowing excess clearance so that no acrylic resin or metal touches the abutments, and a soft reline with tissue conditioner is completed. Preliminary impressions are made with an alginate or hydrocolloid impression material. Interocclusal records are also made at this time.

Laboratory abutment replicas are placed in the impression after making an implant level impression and before pouring in the diestone. The replicas are necessary for determining exact angulation for abutment selection. At this time the mounted casts are used with guide pins in the replicas for diagnostic waxing. Fixture position, angulation, intermaxillary space, smile line, patient expectations, and opposing arch help determine which abutment will be used in the final restoration. Abutment choice will determine the impression technique. Abutment options include the traditional, angulated, EsthetiCone, MirusCone, and UCLA abutments. Wide-platform components are discussed in Chapter 9.

ESTHETICONE ABUTMENT

The EsthetiCone abutment is designed to be used in multple-implant situations if the traditional abutment might cause esthetic compromise with the metal display. It is designed to allow esthetic veneering material to be placed subgingivally, thereby avoiding metal display (Figs. 8-1 and 8-2). The abutment is made of surgical-grade titanium and is available with 1, 2, and 3 mm collars (Fig. 8-3). The depth of the implant determines the size of the abutment that must be used. A gold alloy cylinder and a gold screw are used in the fabrication of the metal frameworks—much the same techniques as described in previous chapters (Fig. 8-4).

The patient is seen 7 to 10 days after abutment surgery. Alginate impressions and an interocclusal registration are made of the maxilla and mandible. The mounted diagnostic casts are used to determine which type of abutment will be used and for fabricating the custom tray. Determination of abutment collar size should not be made until tissue shrinkage after second-stage surgery is complete. At this time the temporary healing abutments are removed, and a periodontal probe is used to measure the distance between the implant and the gingival surface. Abutments are selected individually for each implant to allow 2 mm of veneering material to be

placed subgingivally. Therefore the collar on the abutment should be at least 2 mm below tissue (Figs. 8-5 and 8-6). The abutment is placed in the manual counter-torque device and guided to engage the head of the implant. A light back-and-forth rotation is used to engage the hexagonal portion of the implant (Fig. 8-7). The hexagonal screwdriver is used to tighten the abutment screw (Fig. 8-8). Radiographs are made of the abutments at this time to ensure complete seating. After seating verification, the mechanical or electric torque drivers are used to tighten the abutment screws to 20 Ncm.

Two types of impression copings are available: a square type and a cylindrical type (Figs. 8-9 and 8-10). The square impression is preferred. The impression copings are screwed into place on the abutments using guide pins (Fig. 8-11). An open-window custom tray is placed in the mouth to check for guide pin and coping clearance (Fig. 8-12). After the wax window is placed and the guide pin imprints are captured in wax (as previously described), adhesive is placed, a vinyl polysiloxane or other impression material is mixed, and the impression is made in the usual manner (Fig. 8-13). After the impression material has set, the guide pins are unscrewed until a clicking sound is heard or felt, and the impression is removed. The plastic healing caps are placed on each abutment to prevent tissue collapse (Fig. 8-14). If an interim prosthesis is present, it is relieved and relined with a tissue-conditioning material in the area of the healing caps. An interocclusal record is made at this time.

A cast of the impression can be handled in one of two ways: (1) a small amount of utility wax can be applied around the subgingival area of the impression coping so that the master cast will not fracture upon separation; or (2) tissue conditioner can be painted around the impression coping to

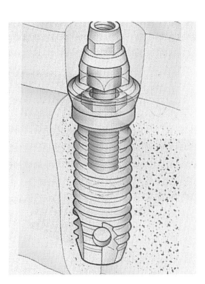

Figure 8-1

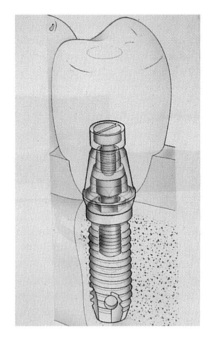

Figure 8-2

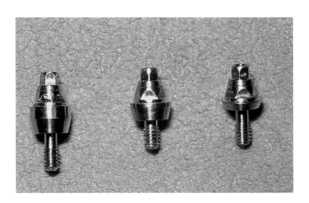

Figure 8-3

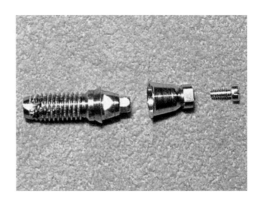

Figure 8-4

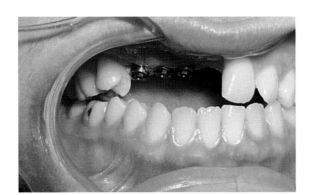

Figure 8-5

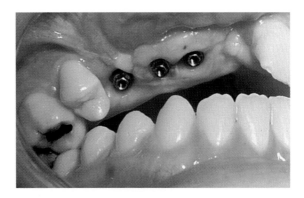

Figure 8-6

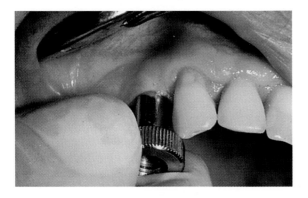

Figure 8-7

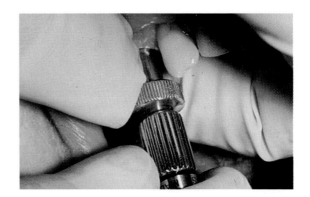

Figure 8-8

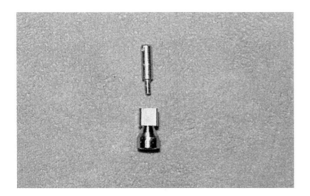

Figure 8-9

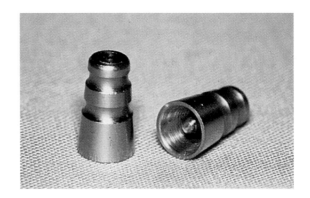

Figure 8-10

simulate the free gingival margin around the abutment (Fig. 8-15). If option 1 is used, the diestone on the lingual side of the abutment is removed to provide access to verify gold cylinder interface seating. Abutment replicas are affixed to the impression coping and secured with guide pins. The impression is cast in diestone, separated, and mounted on a semi-adjustable articulator.

WAXING PROCEDURES

Tapered gold cylinders are placed on the replicas (Fig. 8-16). The casts are closed into centric relation, and the intermax-illary space is measured. A minimum of 6.7 mm is required between the implant flange and the opposing dentition for EsthetiCone components.

Conventional waxing procedures are performed with consideration for the type of veneering material that will be used. Design may include metal, porcelain, or micro-filled composite, depending on the restorative dentist's preference. The wax pattern is sprued, invested, cast, and reclaimed as previously described (Figs. 8-17 to 8-23).

The metal castings are tried in individual units per abutment. One disadvantage with the subgingival margins that

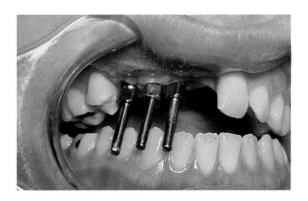

Figure 8-11

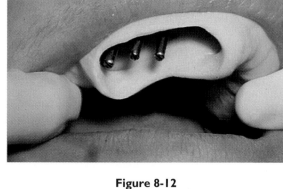

Figure 8-12

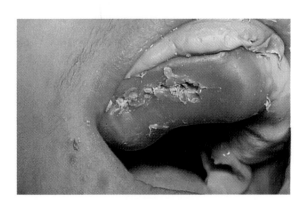

Figure 8-13

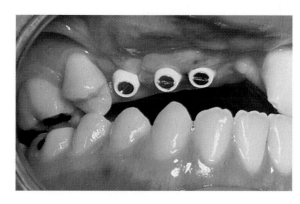

Figure 8-14

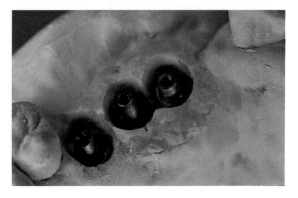

Figure 8-15

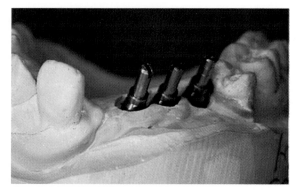

Figure 8-16

exist between the EsthetiCone abutment and prosthetic framework is that the interface accuracy cannot be visualized. Radiograph verification gives a two-dimensional view of the interface, which is affected by radiographic angulation and cannot be verified with complete confidence. Therefore the castings are tried in as individual units (Fig. 8-24). Radiographs are made to evaluate the seating of individual units. Fig. 8-25 shows an example of a distal unit that was incompletely seated because of proximal contact with the adjacent natural tooth. Fig. 8-26 displays radiographic confirmation of the seating after adjustment. Autopolymerizing resin is used for solder indexing, and the castings are removed from the mouth (Fig. 8-27).

Brass replicas are secured to the casting and held in place with guide pins. Undercuts are blocked out with utility wax, and a soldering matrix is constructed from diestone. The casting is placed in a soldering investment, and the soldering is completed (Fig. 8-28).

The healing caps are removed, and the abutments are cleaned of all debris. The hexagonal wrench is used to verify the abutment tightness. The framework is passively tightened on the abutments (Fig. 8-29). The patient is asked if

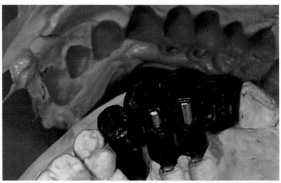

Figure 8-17

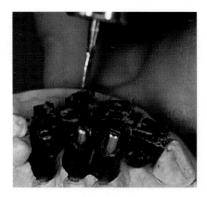

Figure 8-18

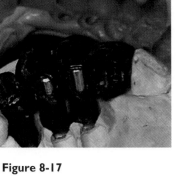

Figure 8-19

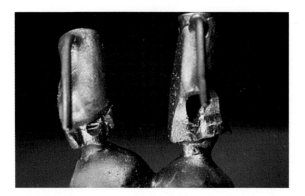

Figure 8-20

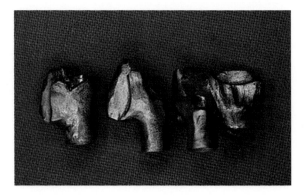

Figure 8-21

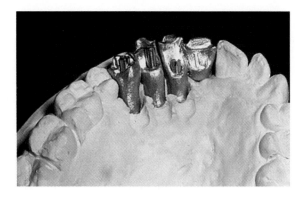

Figure 8-22

any pain exists as the screws are tightened. If pain exists, the patient is requested to differentiate between bony-implant pain and soft-tissue pain. Often the soft tissues may collapse onto the abutment after the healing caps are removed, and the pinching of tissue during framework seating may be painful. Repeated implant pain during the process of tightening and loosening screws indicates that torque is being transmitted into the implants from an ill-fitting frame, or it may indicate that an implant has not integrated. Radiographs are made to examine abutment framework interface (Fig. 8-30). Pain or radiographic evidence of poor fit requires framework sec-

tioning and solder indexing, as previously described. If there is a perfect framework fit, it is ready for veneer application.

The casting is prepared for opaque and porcelain application. Porcelain is applied by conventional methods: contoured, stained, and glazed (Figs. 8-31 and 8-32).

Porcelain application may distort the framework; thus it must be evaluated for fit after porcelain contouring and subsequent porcelain firings. At the delivery appointment, proximal contacts and occlusion are adjusted. The prosthesis is seated, and a radiographic evaluation of fit is completed. The prosthesis is seated onto the abutments, and one of the torque

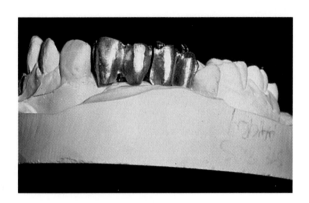

Figure 8-23

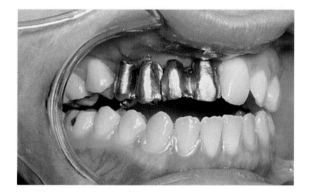

Figure 8-24

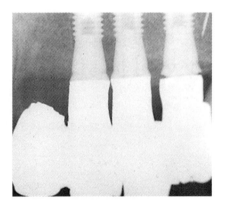

Figure 8-25

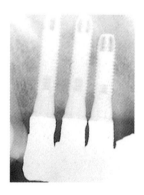

Figure 8-26

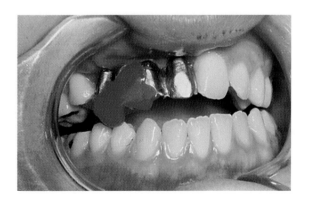

Figure 8-27

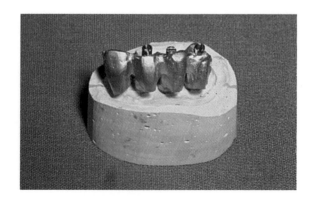

Figure 8-28

drivers is used to tighten the gold screws to 10 Ncm (Figs. 8-33 to 8-35). Temporary restoration material is placed in the screw access holes, and oral hygiene instructions are given to the patient.

PROSTHETIC ATTACHMENT DIRECTLY TO THE IMPLANT (UCLA-TYPE ABUTMENT)

This abutment was originally developed to compensate for space and esthetic limitations that are found with the traditional transmucosal abutment. Combined height of the trans-

mucosal abutment and the gold cylinder left no room for restorative material in certain clinical situations.

Display of the transmucosal abutments in esthetic areas is unacceptable in some clinical situations. The UCLA-type abutment is designed to bypass the transmucosal abutment and fit directly onto the implant (Fig. 8-36). This allows for fabrication of the prosthesis in areas where the intermaxillary space precludes the traditional system. Veneering material can be placed subgingivally, thereby eliminating metal display.

The interface between the implant and abutment is no longer titanium to titanium. Palladium-silver or palladium-

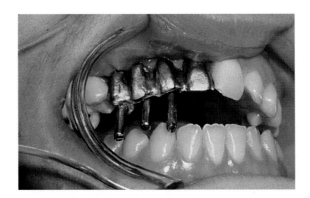

Figure 8-29

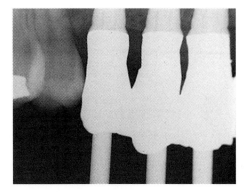

Figure 8-30

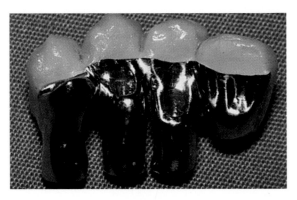

Figure 8-31

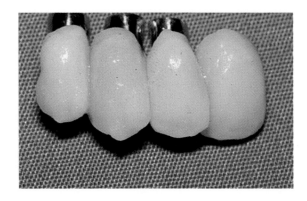

Figure 8-32

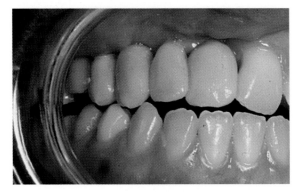

Figure 8-33

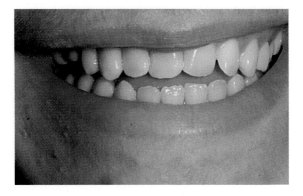

Figure 8-34

gold alloys are most often used in prosthetic framework. Dissimilar metals in contact may produce a galvanic response. This potential galvanic response is located at the implant-framework interface, which is close to the fixture-bone interface. The UCLA-type abutment in its original form was a plastic sleeve that was used as a matrix for waxing and casting the prosthetic framework. A lapping tool with milling paste is used to refine the framework portion of the framework-fixture interface. This is not a controlled machined surface, and because it is located subgingivally it cannot be verified visually. Castings are individual per implant and are indexed in the mouth for soldering.

A lack of intermaxillary space and a metal display with a traditional abutment are indications for use of the UCLA-type abutment (Fig. 8-37).

A premachined cast component is available from Nobel-Biocare. The component is designed to be incorporated into the prosthesis and attaches directly to the implants. This component does not need to be machined like the castable UCLA-type abutment.

PRIMARY IMPRESSIONS

The finished prosthesis bypasses the traditional abutment and fits directly onto the implant. The abutment is removed with the appropriate instrument (Figs. 8-38 and 8-39). Topical anesthetic is placed subgingivally with a cotton pellet.

The pellet is large enough to maintain the diameter of the fixture access and does not allow tissue to collapse. The cotton pellet is removed after 1 minute, and the single-tooth impression coping is placed on the implant; however, the clinician must make sure that the hexagonal head of the implant is engaged. The guide pin is tightened. An impression tray (as previously described) is adapted, and the impression is made. After the guide pins are loosened, the impression is removed, and cotton pellets with topical anesthetic are applied. The abutments are then replaced. An alginate impression of the opposing arch is made, along with an interocclusal record and a facebow transfer.

Pouring the Impressions

The implant replicas are placed on the single-tooth impression coping. The subgingival surface of the single-tooth impression coping should be covered with a light coat of utility wax so that the master cast will not be fractured when it is separated from the impression tray. The master cast is poured in diestone using the usual procedures. Interocclusal records are used to mount the master casts on a semiadjustable articulator. The master cast is prepared by removing the lingual stone at the implant site, exposing the implant replica. This is done to verify the interface between components.

Prostheses are waxed to full contour, allowing access for hygiene. Normal cutback procedures are performed. The

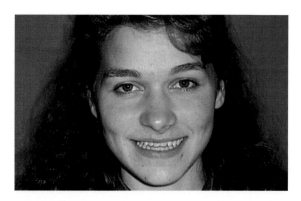

Figure 8-35

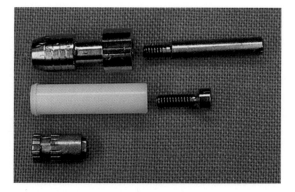

Figure 8-36

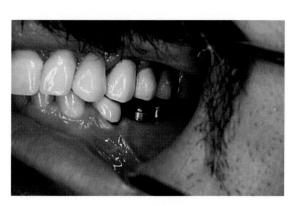

Figure 8-37

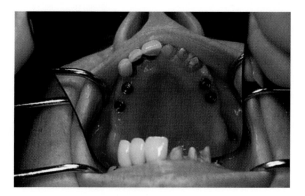

Figure 8-38

interface of the UCLA cylinder will be milled with a lapping procedure after casting unless a premachined component is being used. Each fixture-framework unit is cast in separate pieces or separated before try-in, and a soldering relationship is made in the mouth. The separated wax patterns are individually sprued, invested, cast, and reclaimed.

SOLDERING INDEX

Individual castings are tried intraorally to verify accuracy of fit and to establish a solder matrix. The temporary abutments are removed, topical anesthetic is applied, and individual castings are seated. Adjacent castings are aligned using cuts at the prospective solder joints. Radiographs are made perpendicular to the framework-implant interface to verify the seating. After the seating is verified, a solder index is made using autopolymerizing resin. The framework is removed, and the temporary abutments are replaced.

SOLDERING PROCEDURES

Implant replicas are placed onto the UCLA framework. A soldering index is poured in diestone. The framework is removed, and the self-polymerizing resin is burned off. The individual sections are placed onto the soldering index and luted together. The luted framework is removed from the index and invested in a high-heat soldering investment. Soldering procedures are performed as previously described.

EVALUATING FRAMEWORK FIT

Usual preliminary procedures are performed. Frameworks are seated, and the screws are sequentially tightened. Radiographic verification is completed. The patient is questioned concerning pain around the implants during and after tightening. Soft-tissue discomfort is differentiated from bone discomfort. If interface discrepancy is seen on radiographs or if the patient reports bone pain during or after tightening, the framework is sectioned in the appropriate place, and a new solder index is made.

A combination of buccal porcelain and occlusal light cured resin is used as described in Chapter 4 (Figs. 8-40 to 8-42). The contouring, polishing, and finishing procedures are completed.

CLINICAL SEATING AND DELIVERY

Temporary abutments are again removed, topical anesthetic is applied, and the framework is seated. Proximal contacts are adjusted using disclosing solution. Radiographic verification of seating is accomplished (Figs. 8-43 and 8-44), followed by occlusal adjustment, until the prostheses and adjacent natural teeth hold shimstock (Figs. 8-45 to 8-50). The prosthesis is polished, and screw access holes are temporarily filled. The patient is seen the following day by the hygienist for complete instructions in hygiene. Framework access holes are permanently filled with composite 1 month after seating.

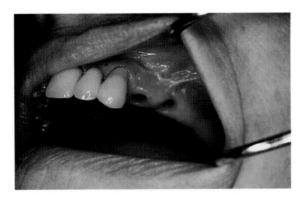

Figure 8-39

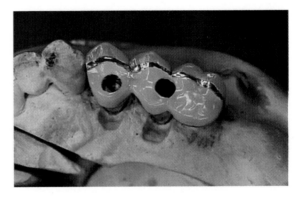

Figure 8-40

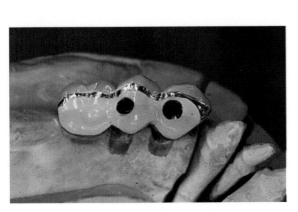

Figure 8-41

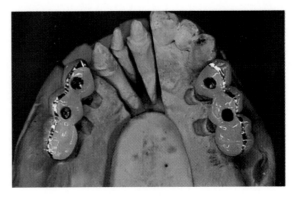

Figure 8-42

DIVERSE ABUTMENT SITUATIONS

Because of implant position and angulation, different abutments may be used in combination in prosthesis design. Lack of intermaxillary space may preclude certain abutments because of component height. In these clinical situations a combination of different abutments is necessary for an acceptable prosthesis result. The patient in Fig. 8-51 had four implants placed in the maxilla. Loss of natural teeth caused supereruption of the opposing mandibular dentition. The distal implant could not be countersunk because of proximity to the maxillary sinus. Fig. 8-52 shows four EsthetiCone

abutments in position. A minimum of 6.7 mm of intermaxillary space is necessary to allow for component height. This space is measured from the head of the implant to the opposing dentition on mounted diagnostic casts. Insufficient space was available for a posterior EsthetiCone or MirusCone abutment. The mandibular crowns were removed, and the occlusal plane was corrected with new crowns. Insufficient space still existed. A UCLA-type abutment that attaches directly to the implant and needs less space was used. Figs. 8-53 to 8-61 show the procedures from impression technique through the finished prosthetics. A diagnostic wax-up during

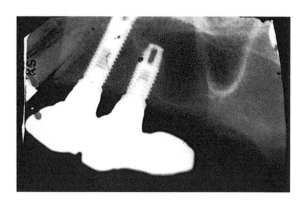

Figure 8-43

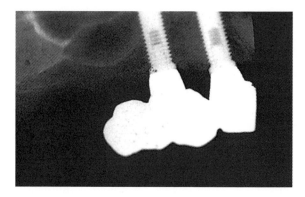

Figure 8-44

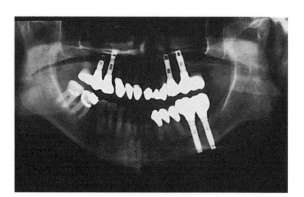

Figure 8-45

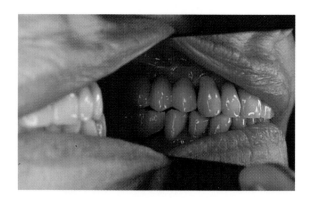

Figure 8-46

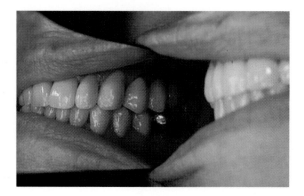

Figure 8-47

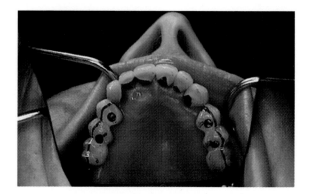

Figure 8-48

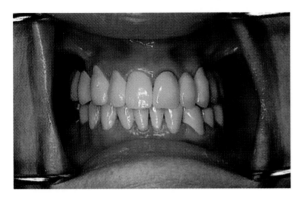

Figure 8-49

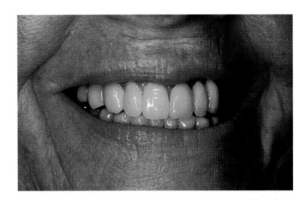

Figure 8-50

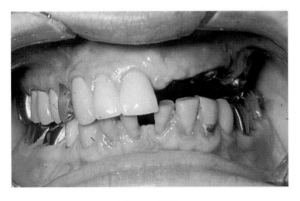

Figure 8-51

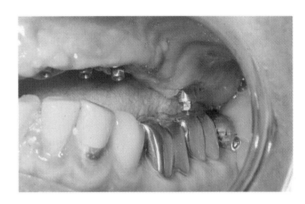

Figure 8-52

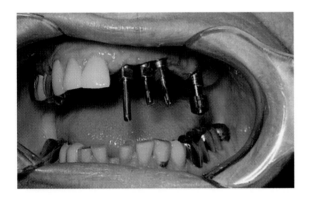

Figure 8-53

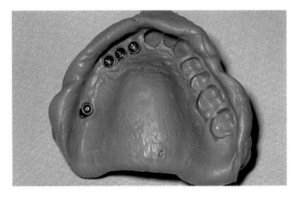

Figure 8-54

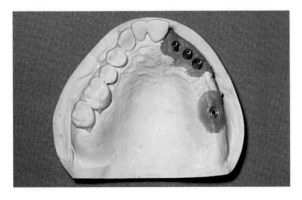

Figure 8-55

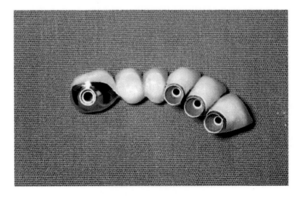

Figure 8-56

treatment planning is the ideal procedure if any question about prosthetic design is presented. Diagnostic impressions made directly on the fixtures allow diagnostic waxing and planning for the proper abutment selection. The waxing before abutment selection saves not only time, but also money.

PARTIALLY EDENTULOUS— UCLA PREPS

Less-than-ideal implant position and angulation may preclude the use of any available abutments in the usual fashion.

Modification of the UCLA-type abutment may compensate for esthetic compromise caused by unfavorable implant position. The patient who is documented had a high smile line complicated by implant position, which would reveal not only a metal display, but would also prevent adequate access for oral hygiene if the available abutments were used in the typical manner (Figs. 8-62 and 8-63). Implant angulation was labial, which produced screw access holes exiting through the facial surface of the prosthetics. Sufficient bone was not available for countersinking the implants. Ideally, implants should be countersunk, placing the implant head at least 4

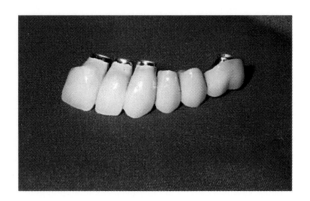

Figure 8-57

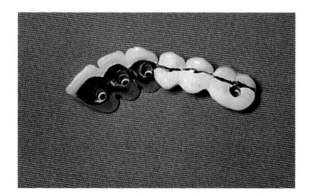

Figure 8-58

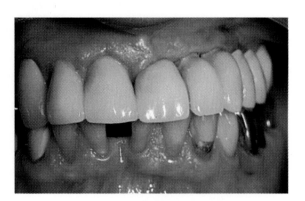

Figure 8-59

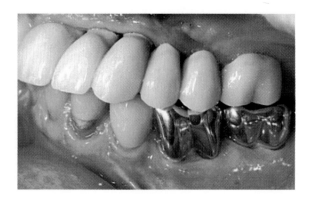

Figure 8-60

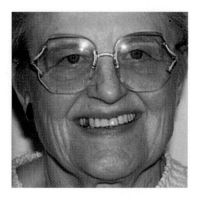

Figure 8-61

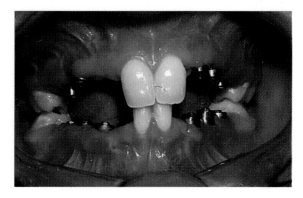

Figure 8-62

mm below tissue. This is especially important in the anterior of the maxilla. The angulated abutment allows for the change of the screw access position, but in this case the angulated abutment collar displayed metal supragingivally, thereby compromising esthetics (Figs. 8-64 and 8-65). Modified UCLA abutments are used to allow acceptable esthetics, along with access for oral hygiene.

Diagnostic casts from impressions made directly on the fixtures are used to determine abutment design (Fig. 8-66). The anterior abutments are designed as telescopic copings using antirotational UCLA-type abutments. The copings are placed in position where the natural tooth abutments are located for ideal esthetics.

From the master cast mounting, nonhexed UCLA-type abutments are placed onto the two most posterior abutments. The anterior hexed antirotational UCLA-type abutments are designed as telescopic preps. The abutments are reduced in length for bite relationship (Figs. 8-67 and 8-68).

A full-contour wax-up is fabricated, and a vinyl polysiloxane matrix is constructed to conform with the facial surfaces using antirotational UCLA-type abutments. Circumferential clearance of the telescopic preps is reverified

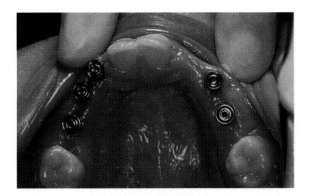

Figure 8-63

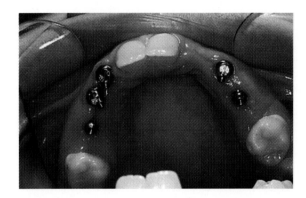

Figure 8-64

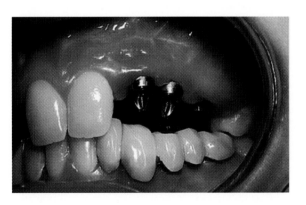

Figure 8-65

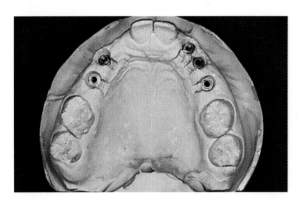

Figure 8-66

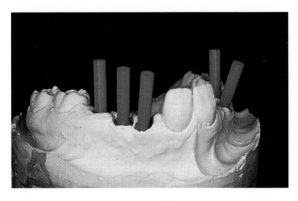

Figure 8-67

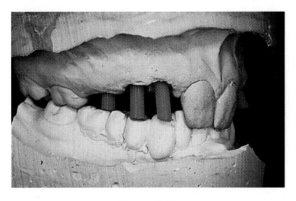

Figure 8-68

by repositioning the matrix on the master cast. The telescopic preps are sprued, invested, cast, reclaimed, and then finished with a lapping procedure performed on the inferior surface of the UCLA abutments to ensure accurate interface between the abutment and implants. The telescopic preps are repositioned into place on the master cast (Figs. 8-69 and 8-70), and the access holes are blocked out with utility wax. A thin coat of wax separator is applied to the preps and surrounding tissue area of the master cast. The matrix is repositioned and held in place with sticky wax. Molten inlay wax is flowed into the matrix and around the preps and is allowed to solidify. The matrix is removed, and the master cast is remounted on the articulator. The bite relationship is verified, and the bridge superstructure is carved and designed, with relieved areas to receive the porcelain. The prosthetic superstructure is designed to be cemented on the copings and screwed directly on the posterior implants using the antirotational UCLA-type abutments (Fig. 8-71); it is sprued, invested, cast, reclaimed, and finished to the telescopic preps and master cast.

After clinical evaluation the prosthetic superstructure is ready for porcelain application. Porcelain is applied, contoured, glazed, and finished (Figs. 8-72 to 8-75).

Figs. 8-76 and 8-77 show anterior modified abutments in position clinically. Radiographs are used to verify complete abutment seating on the implant head. The final prosthesis allows access for oral hygiene. Esthetic compromise caused by the screw access position is eliminated, and metal display is avoided (Fig. 8-78). The Ti-Adapt abutment discussed in Chapter 9 was designed for use in this clinical situation. The computer-generated abutments discussed in Chapter 13 are also appropriate in this situation for abutment design.

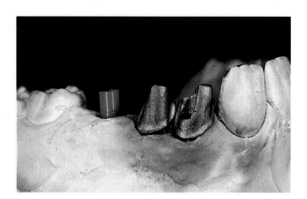

Figure 8-69

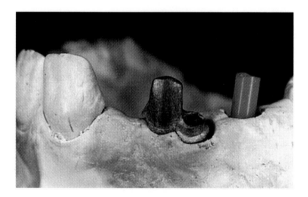

Figure 8-70

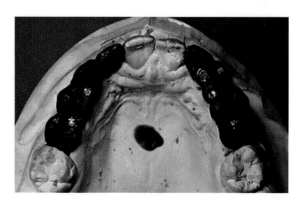

Figure 8-71

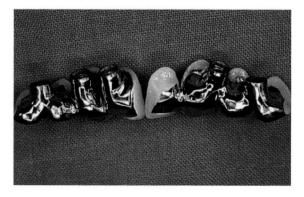

Figure 8-72

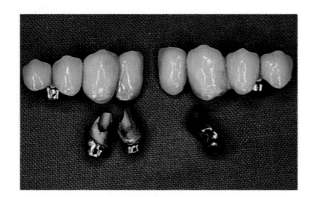

Figure 8-73

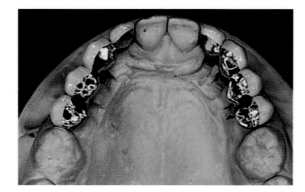

Figure 8-74

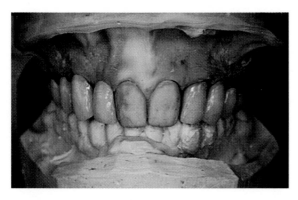

Figure 8-75

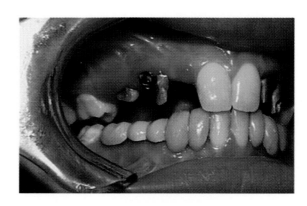

Figure 8-76

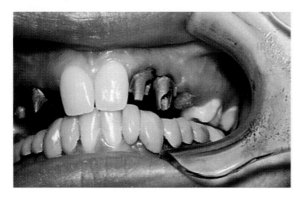

Figure 8-77

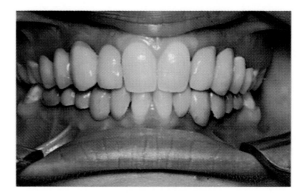

Figure 8-78

Wide-Diameter Implants: Restorative Considerations

Steven G. Lewis

Wide-diameter implants were first developed for the Brane-mark Implant System by Dr. Burton Langer. Langer had several goals in the development of a wider implant. He felt that with greater surface area the wider-diameter implant might be better suited for areas of poor bone quality. In other words, the increase in osseointegration quantity would make up for the decrease in osseointegration quality.

Also, in the posterior region of the mouth where the maxillary sinus or mandibular nerve prevents the placement of a longer implant, a wide-diameter implant could be placed if adequate bone width is present. Thus while the implant is short because of the limited bone height, the added surface area of the wide diameter would make up for the lack of height. In fact, it has been determined that there is as much surface area around a 5.0 mm diameter implant that is 8 mm tall, as there is around a 3.75 mm diameter implant that is 13 mm tall.

Another use of the wide-diameter implant as proposed by Langer was to utilize the implant immediately upon removal of a failed standard-size implant. In other words, if a 3.75 mm diameter implant failed, it could be removed. Then, if adequate healthy bone remained surrounding the failed site, this bone could be immediately prepared for a wider implant. The wide-diameter implant could then be placed into this newly prepared, healthy bone.

Although Langer introduced the wide-diameter implant for the surgical considerations described, the top platform of the 5.0 mm diameter implants had the exact same dimensions as the standard size 3.75 mm diameter and 4.0 mm diameter implants. The size of the external hexagon atop the implant was identical from one implant size to another, and the diameter of the abutment screw channel was identical as well. This made things simple for the restorative dentist since the same transmucosal abutment cylinders and abutment screws would fit either the 3.75 mm, 4.0 mm, or 5.0 mm diameter implants. No matter what diameter implant was present, the same set of abutments could be utilized, and therefore so could the same restorative components. For instance, the same 1 mm EsthetiCone abutment and the corresponding restorative components would fit the 3.75 mm diameter implant, the 4.0 mm diameter implant, and the 5.0 mm diameter implant (Fig. 9-1).

MECHANICAL CONSIDERATIONS

Although the treatment of the edentulous patient with osseointegrated implants has enjoyed tremendous success for over the past 30 years with little need for design changes in implant components, the same cannot be said about the treatment of the partially edentulous patient. Esthetic and functional demands in treating this patient population have required new designs and new techniques. One particular problem in the partially edentulous patient has been the increase in loose and fractured components. To understand why these problems have occurred, one must appreciate the mechanical characteristics of implants and implant components as well as the differences between the edentulous and partially edentulous patient.

When a screw is torqued into position, the stretching of the screw is called *reload*. This reload then creates a clamping force between the two components being held in place. Applied forces that counteract the clamping force will have the potential ability to loosen the screw. Thus if you introduce vertical or axial forces into the implant system, these forces will be well tolerated since they do not act in a way that will separate the components. This is why root-form implants and their various components are designed to tolerate vertical forces exceedingly well. It is lateral forces, or bending, that can be quite destructive as they try to separate the two components being clamped together. If bending moments are constantly applied, there will be a much greater incidence of screw loosening or fracture resulting from the fatigue created over time. The reason that this is not a significant problem in the edentulous patient is because of the tremendous bracing support created by cross-arch splinting. Since the implants are placed across and around the arch, there is a greater chance that any lateral forces introduced to the system will be translated into vertical forces. This is called the *tripod effect* and is similar to sitting on a stool with three legs. If the three legs are well balanced, it is possible to sit on the edge of the stool without tipping over. In the edentulous fixed bridge, bending moments are minimized as a result of this tripod effect. Even if the patient bites on the distal cantilever, introducing bending forces through a fulcrum line between the two most distal implants, the connection of the restoration into all the implants anterior to this fulcrum line provides resistance to the bending, resulting in the forces being more vertical in nature (Fig. 9-2). The greater the curvature of the arch and the more forward the anterior implants are to the fulcrum line, the greater the tripod effect and the greater the resistance to bending. In this scenario the distal cantilevers can be greater. The straighter across the arch the implants are positioned, the less the tripod effect and the less resistance to bending will be present. In this scenario, cantilevering is more dangerous, but in general, the edentulous patient allows for the placement of implants around an arch, providing a good tripod effect and excellent resistance to bending.

When restoring a unilateral quadrant in a partially edentulous patient, the potential benefit of the tripod effect is small. Most mechanical problems have occurred in the posterior region where occlusal forces are great, especially on single- or double-implant restorations where the benefits of tripodding are negligible.

Along with better treatment planning guidelines and more conservative occlusal schemes, it became evident that design changes would be necessary to decrease the problems of bending overload and mechanical fatigue. Wider platforms giving wider bases to the restorations, as well as stronger mechanical components, would be advantageous for improved results.

Using restorations in the posterior mandible as an example, the potential cantilevering and bending is greater buccal-lingual than mesial-distal. With the functional cusp in the posterior mandible being the buccal cusp, in most situations tremendous bending moments are applied during centric occlusal contact. With a normal-size occlusal table, the buccal cusps of an implant restoration are usually beyond the buccal seating surface of the restoration (Fig. 9-3). Therefore when the mandibular buccal cusps come into contact with the opposing tooth or a bolus of food, lateral bending occurs toward the buccal. If a tripod effect with three or more implants is not present to provide resistance to this bending, overload fatigue is possible (Fig. 9-4, A and B). To reduce the bending forces, it is advisable to minimize the buccal-lingual dimension of the occlusal table. The goal is to have the buccal cusp as close as possible to the buccal seating surface of the restoration, minimizing the buccal cantilever.

By increasing the size of the implant platform, bending moments caused by occlusal contacts are decreased (i.e., the buccal cantilever is reduced by the larger platform). The wide-diameter implant developed by Langer was therefore modified so that the top of the implant would contain a wider platform. Today the wide platform implant contains a 5.1 mm diameter top versus 4.1 mm in regular platform implants

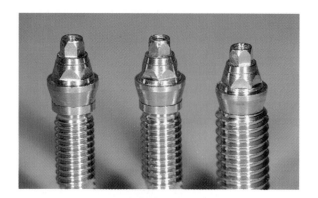

Figure 9-1

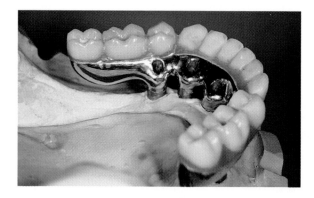

Figure 9-2

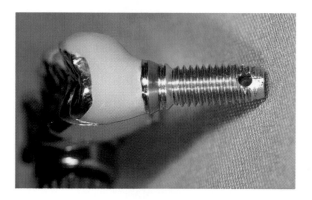

Figure 9-3

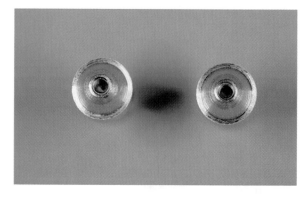

Figure 9-4, A

(Fig. 9-5). Additionally, the abutment screw is 2.5 mm in diameter in the wide platform implant versus 2.0 mm in the regular platform (Fig. 9-6). The larger size of the screw, as well as the ability to create a tighter screw joint, improves the overall strength of the system. The levels of torque applied when tightening the abutment screws are greater, the preload is thus greater, and the clamping force is better. Combined with the wider platform and the resulting decreased potential for bending, this new wide-platform system should withstand the forces of the posterior unilateral implant restoration much greater than before. The result is a design that not only results in less bending overload because

of the wider platforms, but also one that could tolerate increased bending overload because of the stronger screw joints.

RESTORATIVE DESIGN

Several titanium transmucosal abutment designs are available for the wide-platform implant. Single-tooth restorations use the CeraOne WP abutment, whereas multiple-implant restorations utilize MirusCone WP abutments (Fig. 9-7, *A* and *B*). Additionally, the TiAdapt preparable titanium abutments are available for either single-implant or multiple-implant restorations (Fig. 9-8). (*Note*: To distinguish among

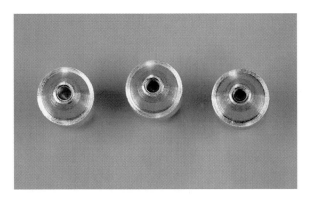

Figure 9-4, B

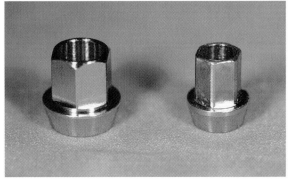

Figure 9-5

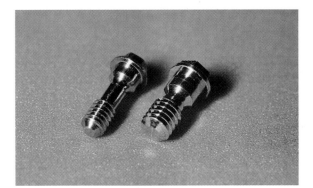

Figure 9-6

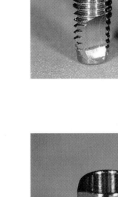

Figure 9-7, A

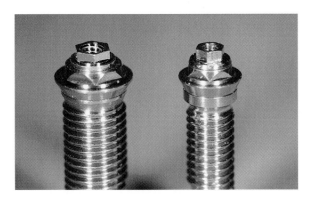

Figure 9-7, B

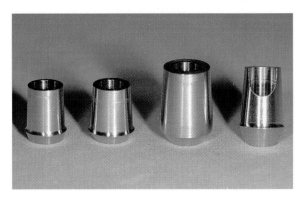

Figure 9-8

the various implant system diameters with the Branemark system, WP, RP, and NP coding is now used: WP denotes wide platform, RP denotes regular platform, and NP denotes narrow platform.)

MULTIPLE-IMPLANT RESTORATIONS (SCREW RETAINED)

MirusCone WP abutments are designed for multiple-implant, screw-retained restorations. They are available with 1 mm, 2 mm, and 3 mm collars. The soft-tissue thickness determines the appropriate collar height. In the posterior region, it is not critical to begin the restoration significantly subgingivally for esthetic reasons, and therefore a collar is selected so as to allow the restoration to begin anywhere from approximately 1 mm beneath the gingival margin to 1 mm above.

The MirusCone abutment is designed for situations where interocclusal distance is minimal but the advantages of a titanium abutment are desired. Since wide-platform implants are to be used in the posterior region where interocclusal limitations are often a concern, the MirusCone is the abutment of choice when determining an appropriate abutment for multiple-implant restorations on the wide-platform implant. A titanium-to-titanium interface is created at the implant/abutment level, a titanium-to–soft tissue interface is created by the collar, and the gingival level of restoration can be controlled by choosing from the three different collar heights. With a 4.2 mm tall gold cylinder, the minimum overall height requirement for restoring the MirusCone WP is 5.2 mm (with the 1 mm collar).

Additionally, the gold-alloy screws that retain the MirusCone WP abutments are tightened with the electric torque controller to 32 Ncm compared with 20 Ncm for the titanium abutment screws on regular-platform implants (see Fig. 9-6). A machine counter-torque protects the system during the tightening process. Again, this larger gold-alloy abutment screw can apply a much stronger clamping force between the abutment and the implant, providing more resistance to any potentially damaging bending moments.

As with other abutment systems designed for screw-retained restorations, the MirusCone WP abutment system includes transfer impression copings, pickup impression copings, laboratory abutment replicas, gold cylinders, and healing caps. The prosthetic gold screw, which contains a hex head and retains the final restoration, is actually strong enough to be tightened to 20 Ncm compared with 10 Ncm for the regular-platform gold screws. This larger and stronger restorative retaining screw provides a stronger clamping force between the restoration and the abutment cylinder.

The restorative seating surface MirusCone WP is 6.0 mm versus 4.8 mm for the MirusCone RP and EsthetiCone RP. Correspondingly, the diameter of the wide-platform gold cylinder is 1.2 mm greater than for the regular-platform gold cylinder (Fig. 9-9). This wider seating surface provides broader support for the restoration and a decreased potential for bending, and it also allows for a more natural restorative appearance (Fig. 9-10). Posterior teeth are wider than anterior teeth, and wide-platform abutments and gold cylinders allow for wider restorations.

Although the wide-platform system, along with its wider platforms and stronger screw joints, are designed to tolerate higher levels of bending forces, it is still advisable to design the occlusion as conservatively as possible. Narrow occlusal tables, centric contacts as close to the centers of the implants as possible, flat occlusal tables, and a lack of lateral occlusal forces all help minimize bending.

A three-implant screw-retained restoration in the posterior mandible using the wide-platform components is illustrated in Fig. 9-11, *A* to *F*.

MULTIPLE-IMPLANT RESTORATIONS (CEMENT RETAINED)

For clinicians who prefer to fabricate cement-retained restorations, the Branemark Implant System provides the TiAdapt abutment system (see Fig. 9-8). These titanium abutments are screw retained to the implants and allow for the implant restoration to be cement retained rather than screw retained. The abutments must be first prepared to the desired

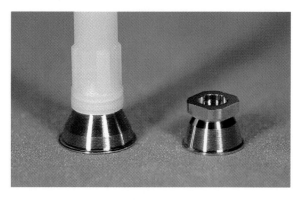

Figure 9-9

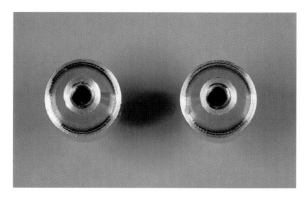

Figure 9-10

configurations. Standard crown and bridge procedures are then performed for impressions and delivery.

One advantage of prepared abutments is the ability to design the restorative margin to parallel soft-tissue contour. This is more critical for cement-retained restorations then for screw-retained restorations because screw-retained restorations usually involve prefabricated machined components that provide for extremely small gaps between the restoration and the abutment. Cement-retained restorations usually result in larger gaps, especially when waxing and casting the restoration rather then using prefabricated components, and these larger gaps can cause considerable harm when they are

too far subgingival. Removing excess cement at the restorative margin is also much more difficult when this margin is excessively subgingival. Proper preparation of an abutment based on the gingival contours should make the cement removal much easier.

A concern with cementable restorations is that retrievability can be much more difficult. If the abutment screw loosens and the cement retention remains intact, it could be difficult to retrieve the restoration in order to gain access to the abutment screw. For this reason, the abutment screw in the TiAdapt system is designed to provide an extremely strong joint. The gold-alloy abutment screw for the regular-platform

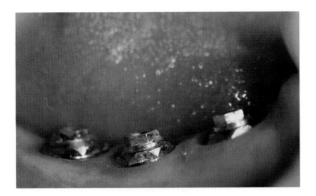

Figure 9-11, A

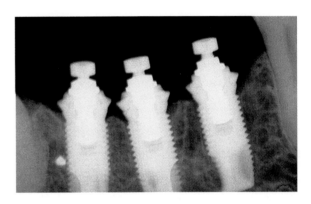

Figure 9-11, B

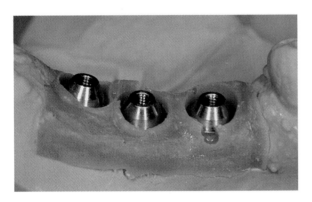

Figure 9-11, C

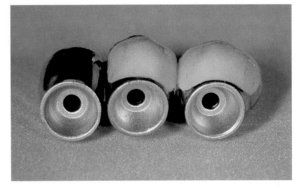

Figure 9-11, D

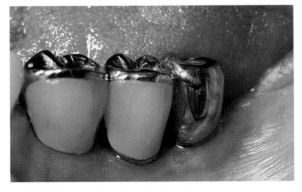

Figure 9-11, E

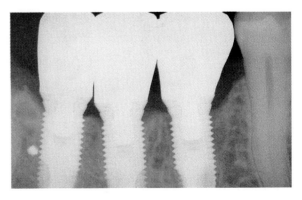

Figure 9-11, F

series is tightened 32 Ncm, whereas the abutment screw for the wide-platform series is tightened to 45 Ncm (Fig. 9-12). Counter-torque is necessary for either series.

A double-implant cement-retained restoration on one wide-platform and one regular-platform implant is illustrated in Fig. 9-13, *A* to *H*.

SINGLE-IMPLANT RESTORATIONS

The wide-platform implant can be used for single-tooth replacement with the CeraOne WP abutment (see Fig. 9-7, *B*). As with CeraOne RP and CeraOne NP abutments, the CeraOne WP abutment is designed for cement-retained restorations. The CeraOne WP abutment is available with 1 mm, 2 mm, and 3 mm collars. The diameter of the collar forming the restorative base is 6.0 mm compared with 4.8 mm for the CeraOne RP. The restoration therefore has a 1.2 mm wider base, providing for more stability (less potential for bending) and improved esthetics in the posterior region where teeth are generally wider. Either a gold cylinder (4.7 mm tall) or burnout pattern can be used to create the final porcelain-fused-to-metal or all-metal restoration (Fig. 9-14). The impression coping, healing cap, temporary cap,

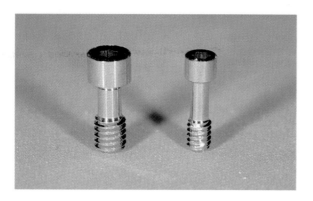

Figure 9-12

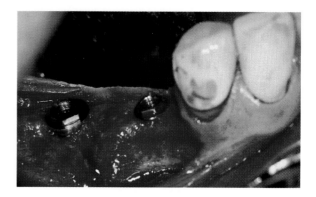

Figure 9-13, A

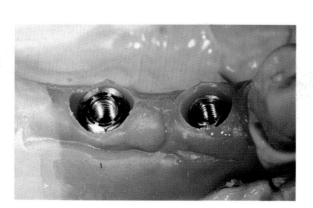

Figure 9-13, B

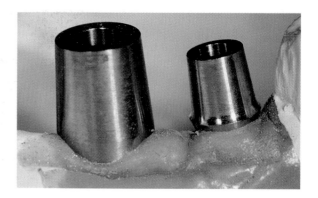

Figure 9-13, C

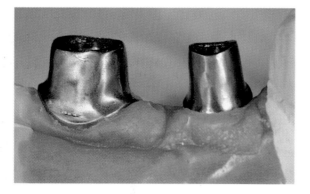

Figure 9-13, D

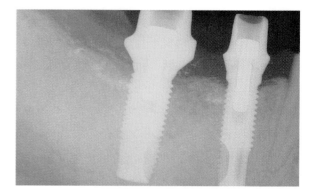

Figure 9-13, E

and laboratory abutment replica are simply wider versions of the regular-platform series and are used in a similar fashion.

The gold-alloy abutment screw is similar in width to the MirusCone WP abutment screw (2.5 mm wide compared with 2 mm for the regular-platform abutment screws). The CeraOne WP abutment screw can actually be tightened to 45 Ncm with the electric torque controller. A machine counter-torque device is necessary to avoid damaging the fixture-to-bone anchorage during this procedure. The final result is an extremely strong screw joint.

TREATMENT PLANNING CONSIDERATIONS

Although the wide-platform implant system does have advantages both surgically and restoratively, its use in certain situations may be contraindicated. For instance, if a wide-diameter implant is placed in the anterior region where buccal-lingual bone dimension may be marginal, do the advantages of the wide-platform implant outweigh the potential harm of leaving inadequate bone around the implant? To compare this situation with a more familiar dental scenario, do the benefits of widening a post outweigh the disadvantage of overly weakening the tooth? There is a tendency today in implant dentistry to think that if the wide-diameter implant has advantages over standard-diameter implants, then it

should be used whenever possible. This thinking is based more on a mechanical level then on a biologic level. The implant and restoration must ultimately be supported by bone, a living tissue. Without adequate bone support, the advantages of a stronger pillar could be overshadowed by osseointegration failure. It has been found in restorative dentistry that longer posts are much more beneficial than wider posts when it comes to the health of the surrounding tissues (the tooth).

Now that osseointegrated implants have been used in the partially edentulous patient long enough to provide lessons from failure, knowledge is available to help determine when it might be beneficial to reduce the amount of bone for the sake of wider components versus preserving as much bone as possible and using more standard-size components. For instance, some compromises have been seen when molar restorations are supported by single implants (Fig. 9-15). On occasion, the wide occlusal table may be too wide for the supporting implant and the resulting bending moments cause complications with the restorative components, the bone implant interface, or the integrity of the implant itself. Today one would certainly consider the use of a wide-diameter implant, as well as wider and stronger restorative components, for the fabrication of an implant-supported single-molar restoration. However, problems with single

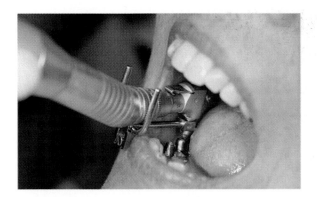

Figure 9-13, F

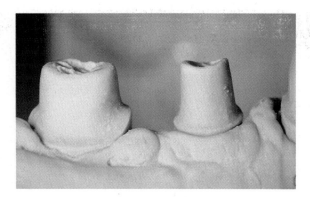

Figure 9-13, G

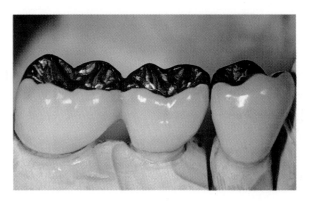

Figure 9-13, H

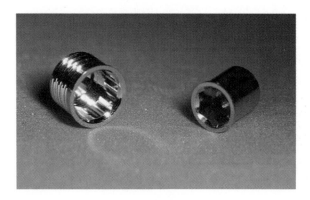

Figure 9-14

anterior teeth supported by implants have not occurred to an extent that would cause one to consider removing additional bone for the sake of a wider implant. Therefore the use of wider-diameter implants posteriorly for single-tooth restorations can be argued but would be difficult to justify in the anterior region.

For multiple-implant restorations there have been complications in the posterior region when the restoration is supported by two implants. The problems are possibly due to the bending moments created by either lateral forces or axial forces cantilevered too far buccally or lingually. As previously stated, the placement of a third implant and the establishment of a tripod effect is a tremendous advantage compared with two implants, but sometimes it is not possible to place a third implant. In these situations the use of wide-diameter implants may be beneficial. With wider seating surfaces for the restoration there is less bending overload. With narrow occlusal tables and wide-diameter implants, it is possible to minimize buccal or lingual bending dramatically. Three standard-diameter implants are still optimal because of the tre-mendous resistance to bending as well as preserving max-

imum bone around each implant, but if only two implants can be placed and adequate bone is present, two wide-diameter implants are definitely an advantage over two standard-diameter implants (Fig. 9-16, *A* and *B*). Therefore, in the replacement of two molars when it is not possible to bicuspidize one of the molars for the placement of three implants, two wide-diameter implants would be the treatment of choice. If a premolar and molar are to be placed and only two implants are planned, two wide-diameter implants may again be advantageous; however, in the premolar region the use of a wide-diameter implant may jeopardize the quantity of the surrounding bone. In this case perhaps a standard-diameter implant could be used in the position of the second premolar while a wide-diameter implant is placed in the first molar site.

There is no doubt that decisions concerning implant size should be made on a case-by-case basis. In general, however, it could be stated that wide-diameter implants should at least be considered for all single- or double-implant restorations in the molar region to maximize the chance for success and minimize the potential for maintenance problems.

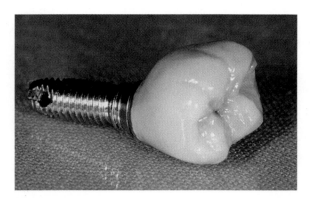

Figure 9-15

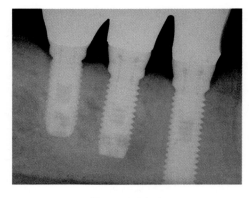

Figure 9-16, A

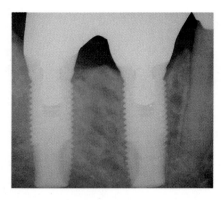

Figure 9-16, B

Implant-Assisted Overdentures

An implant-retained overdenture is an alternative form of treatment to the fixed-implant prosthesis. The overdenture is retained by one of many types of mechanical retention. The denture may attach on a cast bar fixed to the abutments, or it may attach to individual abutments. The patient can remove the overdenture for cleaning. Unconnected abutments and the smaller configuration of the attachment bar (in comparison with the fixed implant prosthesis) allow a simplified hygiene protocol.

Patients who have worn conventional dentures for many years and have undergone extensive ridge resorption may require an overdenture to provide acceptable tissue support. The position of the distal-most implant limits the cantilever extension with the fixed-implant prosthesis. Patients may not accept the tissue support provided by second premolar or first molar extensions. The overdenture extensions can provide desired tissue support while allowing first- or second-molar occlusion. Fewer implants, abutments, and prosthetic components are required for an overdenture, greatly lowering the cost for treatment. Other advantages include less component stress and breakage and a simplified technique in most situations. When trauma or resorption has diminished the alveolar process in the maxilla, the overdenture may be more esthetic than the fixed prosthesis becaused of better facial contours provided by the denture flange.

DISADVANTAGES

Attachments wear with repeated removal and seating of the overdenture. Biting the attachment denture to place may distort or break attachments. Bone resorption is slowed or stopped by implants, stimulating the bone around implants, but changes in tissue support for overdentures must be monitored, and periodic relines are needed for most patients. Costs for maintaining overdentures may offset the lower initial cost of treatment compared with a fixed prosthesis.

Disadvantages also include potential movement and irritation from a removable prosthesis or psychological problems associated with a removable prosthesis.

TREATMENT PLANNING

Panoramic radiographs and mounted diagnostic casts are made; intraoral, head, and neck examinations are completed; and an in-depth patient interview is performed. During examination, existing dentures are evaluated for vertical dimension of occlusion, lip and cheek support, and esthetics. Models of prosthetic options and pictures or slides of patients with different prosthetic options are shown. The patient's opinion of tissue support, specifically nasolabial fold, is explored. If the existing labial flange is necessarily thick to compensate for resorption or if the patient's expectations for tissue support include excess support in this area, then an overdenture is indicated, unless a bone graft is used (Figs. 10-1 to 10-3). The buccal corridor and tooth display in the existing prosthesis are evaluated. A patient who shows first or second maxillary molars during maximum smiling may have an unacceptable gap with the fixed-implant prosthesis because of limited cantilever allowed in the maxilla. An overdenture is indicated in this situation also. After prosthetic evaluation and consultation, the patient is referred for surgical evaluation. After consultations with the surgeon and the restorative dentist, discussions about the availability of bone for implant placement, and discussions concerning the patient's expectations in light of financial realities, a decision can be reached concerning prosthetic options.

MANDIBLE

Tissue support in the mental labial fold and external oblique region is evaluated. Patient expectations are discussed. Models of different options are shown, including overdentures with various retentive and financial options, as well as the fixed-implant prosthesis. Pictures of patients with different prosthetic options may be helpful also.

As the patient handles the various models and removes and replaces the dentures, finger strength and dexterity can be evaluated. Examinations, radiographs, records, and surgical evaluations use the same procedures as those used with the maxillary overdenture.

OVERDENTURE OPTIONS

Bar Attachment Systems

1. Mechanical
   a. Clips
   b. Stud
   c. O-rings
2. Magnetic

Unconnected Fixture Options

1. Mechanical
   a. Magnetic

The bar attachment system for retaining the overdenture distributes functional force to all implants. More retentive options are available with the cast bar. A number of attachments are available, and most work well if used properly. More than one attachment per implant may be used with a bar system; only one attachment per implant is possible if no bar is used to connect implants. The bar attachment systems require more components and higher laboratory expense and may be more technique sensitive. Moderate dexterity is necessary for hygiene and placement and removal of the overdenture. Position and number of implants will dictate the length and distal extension of the bar, as well as the number of attachments used. With four or more implants the bar may be cantilevered 10 mm distal to the distal-most implants, allowing an overdenture, which is mainly implant-supported in the mandible. Fewer implants require a combination of tissue and implant support. In the maxilla, four or more implants will allow three or more attachments on the bar and elimination of full palatal coverage. The final denture may have the majority of palatal acrylic removed, leaving the overdenture in a horseshoe configuration.

PROCEDURES—MAXILLA AND MANDIBLE

Impression procedures are similar to those described for the fixed-implant–supported prosthesis. Preliminary alginate impressions are made 2 weeks after second-stage surgery. The denture is relieved in the area of the abutments and relined with a tissue-conditioning material. Custom trays are fabricated with vestibular and palatal extensions similar to a complete denture. The open-window design is used. After complete healing the final impression is made. The titanium hemostats and hexagonal wrench are used to verify abutment tightness. Occasionally, the abutments may appear tight and seated but are not completely seated on the hexagonal head of the implant. Loosening and retightening the abutment or a radiographic verification can determine the seating. All plaque and calculus are removed from the abutments, and the impression copings are placed (Figs. 10-4 and 10-5). The custom tray is border molded, baseplate wax is used to seal the window, and the tray is placed in the mouth to capture guide pin positions in the wax (Figs. 10-6 and 10-7). After adhesive use, the final impression is made. The tray is filled and is seated completely over the guide pins and the impression copings, and border molding is completed (Fig. 10-8). The guide pins are loosened, and the impression is removed. The laboratory replicas are placed, and the impression is poured in diestone as previously described

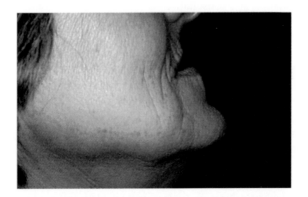

Figure 10-1

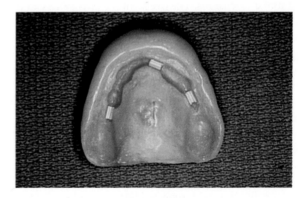

Figure 10-2

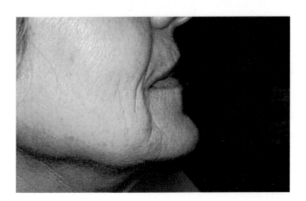

Figure 10-3

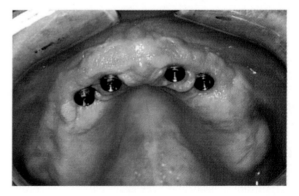

Figure 10-4

(Figs. 10-9 and 10-10). The attachment and bar extensions are discussed with the laboratory.

Depending on the treatment plan, several clipbar attachments may be considered for the prosthesis, such as a precast clipbar, a Dolder bar, or a plastic custom pattern (Hader bar and CBS System). Additional attachments include stud overdenture attachments, such as Sterngold's ERA, O-SO, and Nobelpharma's ball attachment. Attachments are incorporated into the wax pattern design of the bar, sprued, invested, cast, and reclaimed in the normal manner (Figs. 10-11 to 10-15).

The casting is evaluated for fit on the abutments. The healing caps are removed, and the abutments are cleaned of all calculus and plaque. The hexagonal wrench is used to tighten the abutments. The attachment bar is passively screwed in place. The framework-abutment interface is checked for accuracy as previously described (Fig. 10-16). The bar is sectioned and soldered if necessary. When an accurate fit exists, a processed base can be made.

PROCESSED BASE

A processed base incorporating attachments provides several advantages when compared with traditional baseplate use. The processed base snaps into the attachment bar, providing stability for interocclusal records. Denture soreness can be

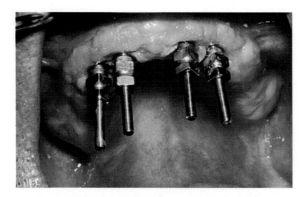

Figure 10-5

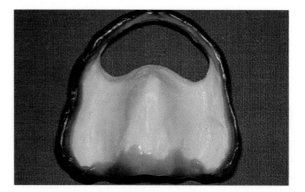

Figure 10-6

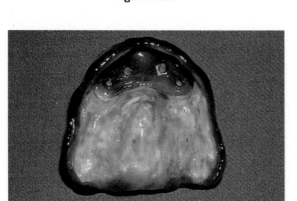

Figure 10-7

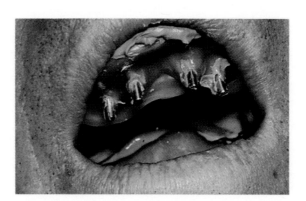

Figure 10-8

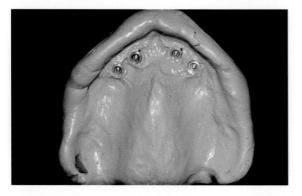

Figure 10-9

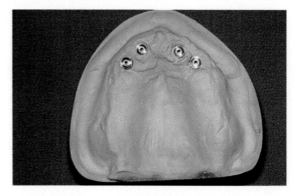

Figure 10-10

adjusted before delivery of the completed prosthesis. Fit and retention from attachments can be perfected before delivery also.

The bar is placed on the master cast with gold screws. Laboratory analogues are placed in each attachment (Figs. 10-17 and 10-18). Fast-set plaster is mixed and flowed over the bar, leaving the analogues exposed. The plaster is contoured to completely cover the bar with no undercuts. The minimum amount of plaster to accomplish this is used. Two thicknesses of baseplate wax are placed onto the master cast (Fig. 10-19), extending over normal denture extensions. The cast is invested in the usual manner and processed with den-

ture acrylic. After processing, the denture and bar are carefully retrieved from the plaster. The attachment bar is separated from the attachments in the processed base; it is then snapped back into the base to evaluate retention and complete the seating of attachments. The base is trimmed and polished (Fig. 10-20). A wax occlusion rim is then added (Fig. 10-21).

MAXILLOMANDIBULAR RELATIONS

The attachment bar is positioned in the mouth. Pressure indicator paste is placed on the internal area of the processed base and is seated in the mouth. Attachment retention is

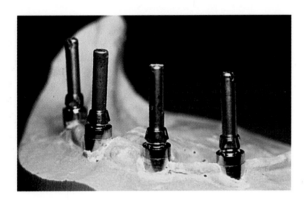

Figure 10-11

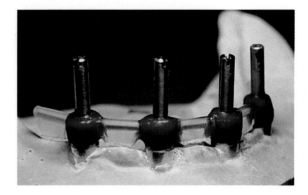

Figure 10-12

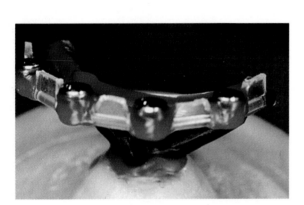

Figure 10-13

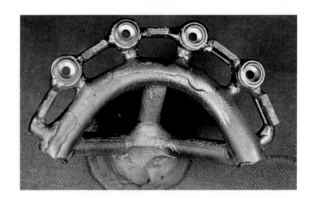

Figure 10-14

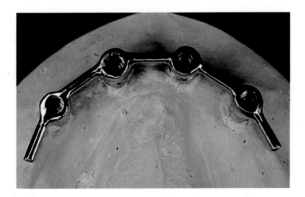

Figure 10-15

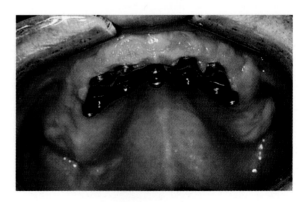

Figure 10-16

checked, as is potential denture soreness. If attachments are not seated, denture acrylic in the region of the bar may prevent seating. Examination of the pressure indicator paste pattern and adjustment will allow complete seating. After complete seating has occurred, maxillomandibular relations are completed, establishing lip support and phonetics at the proper vertical dimension of occlusion. Centric relation records and facebow transfer are completed (Figs. 10-22 and 10-23).

The baseplate is mounted on a semiadjustable articulator. Condylar settings are made (if appropriate). Wax contours that are established during maxillomandibular relations are used as guidelines for tooth arrangement.

The bar is secured in the patient's mouth, and the trial tooth arrangement is evaluated (Fig. 10-24). Esthetics, phonetics, and the vertical dimension of occlusion are evaluated. When all parameters are acceptable, another centric relation record is made. Denture soreness can again be adjusted during this appointment.

The denture is processed in the usual manner. After processing, breakout, and laboratory occlusal adjustment have occurred, the overdenture is again snapped into the attachment bar. Occasionally during processing, acrylic may flow into the attachment areas. The acrylic is adjusted again to allow complete seating of the overdenture into the attach-

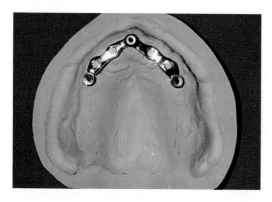

Figure 10-17

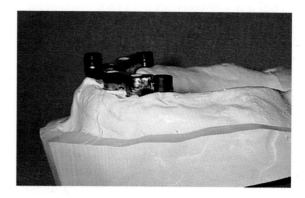

Figure 10-18

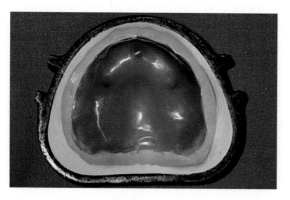

Figure 10-19

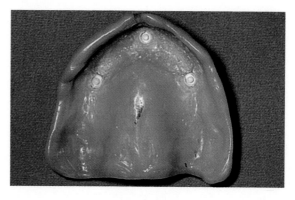

Figure 10-20

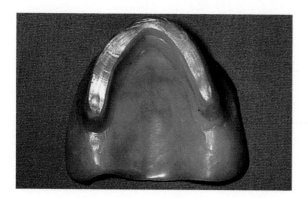

Figure 10-21

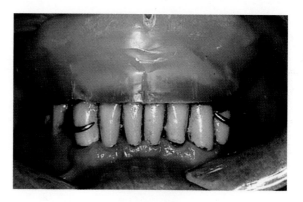

Figure 10-22

ment bar. The denture is then polished. The palatal portion of the maxillary denture may be removed if four or more fixtures are present.

CLINICAL DELIVERY

The denture is again snapped onto the attachment bar (Figs. 10-25 and 10-26). Pressure indicator paste is used to adjust potential denture soreness. A centric relation record is made, and the denture is remounted in the laboratory for final occlusal refinement. The torque wrench is used to tighten all gold screws to 10 Ncm. Hygiene and homecare instructions are given at this time also.

MANDIBULAR OVERDENTURE CLIPBAR—TWO-FIXTURE, TISSUE-SUPPORTED, USING A PRECAST NOBELPHARMA CLIPBAR OR A DOLDER BAR

From a technical and economical standpoint, several advantages are realized when using this system. Technically speaking the system is one of the least complicated because it is a simple technique involving two solder joints that connect the bar to the gold cylinders. The kit consists of two gold cylinders, two gold screws, a gold bar, and two clip retainers (Fig. 10-27).

SETUP AND SOLDERING

The gold cylinders are placed onto the abutment replicas and secured into place with guide pin screws (Fig. 10-28). The bar is placed between the two gold cylinders (Fig. 10-29). The precast bar is cut to the required length (Fig. 10-30). The bar is positioned between the cylinders and secured into place with either sticky wax or cyanoacrylate adhesive (Fig. 10-31). The guide pins are unscrewed, and the bar assembly is removed from the master cast and positioned into a soldering investment. Basic soldering techniques are performed using the manufacturer's recommended solder (Fig. 10-32). The bar is reclaimed from the investment, cleaned, rubber wheeled, and polished, using protective measures that will not damage the inferior surface of the gold cylinders (Fig. 10-33).

The completed clipbar is returned to the clinic for a try-in to verify accuracy intraorally. An inaccurate fit requires sectioning, indexing, and resoldering the bar (Fig. 10-34).

OVERDENTURE PROCESSING TO NOBELPHARMA CLIPBAR

The clipbar is placed on the master cast and held in position with gold screws. The two retentive clips are evenly spaced on the bar between the gold cylinders (Fig. 10-35). The bar and the gold cylinders are blocked out with dental plaster (Fig. 10-36); the overdenture wax-up is repositioned on the cast,

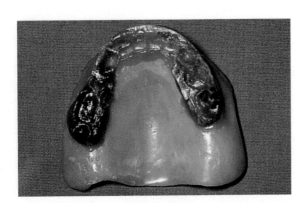

Figure 10-23

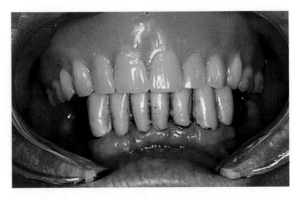

Figure 10-24

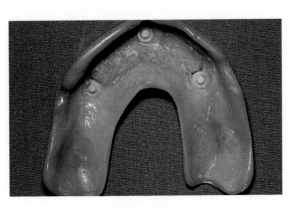

Figure 10-25

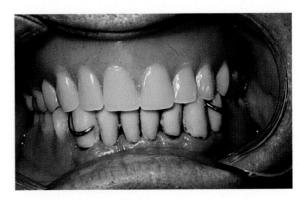

Figure 10-26

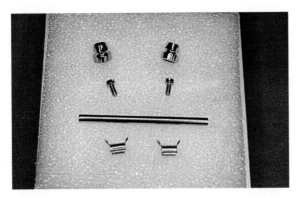

Figure 10-27

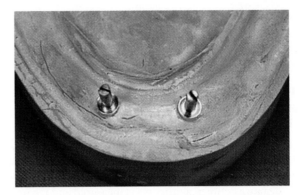

Figure 10-28

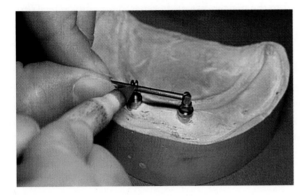

Figure 10-29

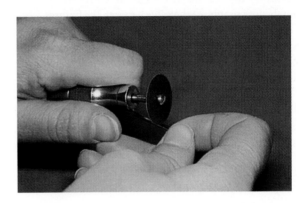

Figure 10-30

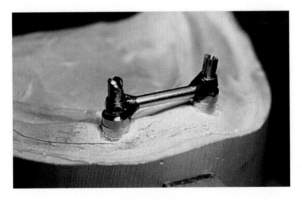

Figure 10-31

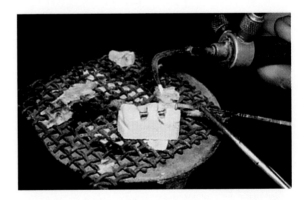

Figure 10-32

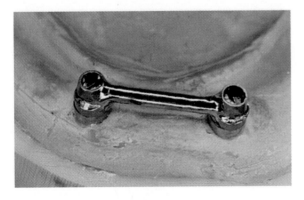

Figure 10-33

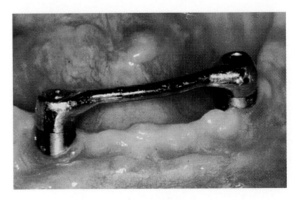

Figure 10-34

sealed, and processed in the normal manner. The overdenture is finished and polished; clip retention is verified on the master cast (Figs. 10-37 and 10-38), and they are returned to the clinic for delivery.

MANDIBULAR OVERDENTURE CLIPBAR—PREFABRICATED PLASTIC CLIPBAR PATTERN

A 1 mm thickness of inlay wax is flowed around the retentive surface of gold cylinder. The cylinders are placed on the brass abutment replicas and are held in place with guide pin screws. The distance between abutments is measured and recorded, and the prefabricated plastic bar is cut to proper length. The inferior borders of the plastic bar are trimmed to conform with the topography of the ridge between the fixtures. The bar is aligned with the retromolar pads and is relieved sufficiently so that it does not rest on the tissue, thereby minimizing the possibility of tissue hyperplasia occurring in the future, yet allowing adequate space for hygiene maintenance.

The bar is then secured into position with cyanoacrylate adhesive or sticky wax. Adequate dimension must be maintained for strength in the connecting joints' different proportions.

An indirect spruing technique is preferred for this clipbar because it adds rigidity and support for the assembled pattern. An 8-gauge wax sprue is placed on the lingual surface of each gold cylinder. To ensure the integrity of the retentive surface of the bar, a third sprue is attached to the inferior lingual surface of the plastic bar. A 6-gauge, plastic, wax-coated feeder bar is placed and secured to the sprued bar. Two 6-gauge wax feeder sprues then are attached to the bar, the guide pins are removed, and the assembled sprued pattern is weighed to determine the amount of alloy that will be needed for the casting. The pattern is placed on a sprue former and is vacuum invested using a phosphate investment. Burnout and casting procedures are performed to the manufacturer's directions. The clipbar is cast, reclaimed, cleaned, fit evaluated to the master cast, and prepared for clinical trial fitting.

MANDIBULAR OVERDENTURE CLIPBAR
Three- or Four-Implant Supported

The advantages of the implant-supported clipbar include the overdenture being secured to the bar at three or four positions, thereby giving at least a tripod retention configuration (Fig. 10-39). This design can produce great stability in

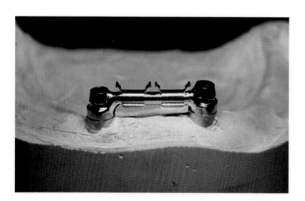

Figure 10-35

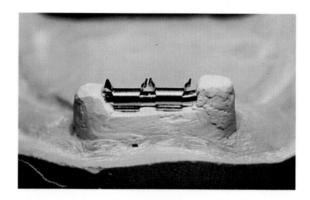

Figure 10-36

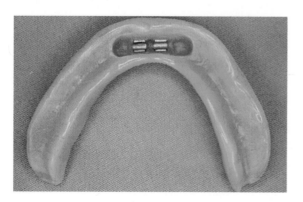

Figure 10-37

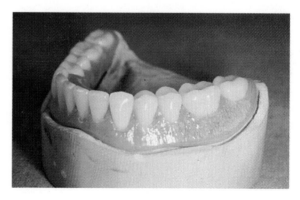

Figure 10-38

the final prosthesis by using either a clipbar or stud attachments, or a combination of the two.

The retentive plastic clip is 5 mm wide; therefore to allow adequate room, a 7 to 8 mm plastic pattern is cut for the distal extensions. The distal extended patterns are secured with extreme caution to the gold cylinders along the crest of the ridge.

An indirect spruing technique is the method of preference for the clipbar, adding rigidity and support for the assembled pattern. An 8-gauge wax sprue is placed on the lingual surface of each gold cylinder. To ensure the integrity of the retentive surface of the bar, a third sprue is attached to the inferior lingual surface of the plastic bar. A 6-gauge, plastic, wax-coated feeder bar is placed and secured to the sprued bar. Two 6-gauge wax feeder sprues are attached to the bar, the guide pins are removed, and the assembled sprued pattern is weighed to determine the amount of alloy required for the casting. The pattern is placed on a sprue former and is vacuum invested, using a high-heat phosphate investment. Burnout and casting procedures are performed to the manufacturer's directions.

The clipbar is cast, reclaimed, and cleaned; the fit is evaluated on the master cast. The clipbar is finished and polished.

When the clipbar fit has been verified, the overdenture is processed and finished in the usual manner. (Figs. 10-40 to 10-43).

OVERDENTURE CLIPBAR—THREE TO FOUR FIXTURES WITH EXTRACORONAL ATTACHMENTS

The implant-assisted overdenture is an alternative to the maxillary and the mandibular fixed bridge. The prosthetic design has a number of advantages. Because of underlying bone resorption the extra bulk in the overdenture creates more facial tissue support. The patient's hygiene maintenance is easier because the removal of the overdenture allows greater access for cleaning. In some cases the palate in the maxillary overdenture may be removed to enable the patient to have a greater thermal sensitivity and increased taste sensation.

The impressions for the clipbars are taken in the usual manner with open-windowed custom trays. Impression copings and guide pins are placed, and the tissue is impressed using vinyl polysiloxane impression material. Clinical and laboratory procedures are similar to those shown in Figs. 10-4 to 10-26.

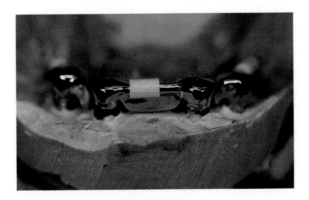

Figure 10-39

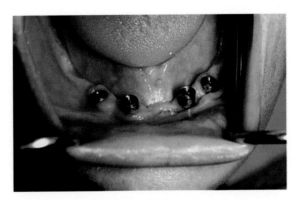

Figure 10-40

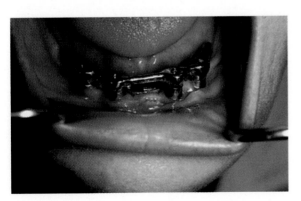

Figure 10-41

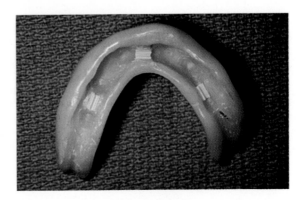

Figure 10-42

LABORATORY PROCEDURES

The master casts are poured and mounted on a semiadjustable articulator using the intraoral bite registrations. The gold cylinders are secured to the abutment replicas with guide pin screws. Inlay wax is placed around each gold cylinder, and wax is flowed to connect each of the cylinders, forming a wax bar.

Two ERA extracoronal attachments and two O-SO attachments are affixed to the bar waxing using a surveyor for parallelism. The two extracoronal attachments are placed distal to the posterior abutments on the crest of the ridge. When waxing the inferior surfaces, adjacent space must be allowed for proper hygiene.

On the mandible (Figs. 10-44 to 10-49), two ERA extracoronal attachments, along with two O-SO rings, are used. The O-SO attachments were chosen because of the lack of distance they have between the abutments. This distance does not allow for ERAs or clipbar design.

Waxing is similar to that stated previously for the clipbar procedures, with the parallel placement of the O-SO attachments on the superior surface (as shown).

The wax patterns are directly sprued and cast in a normal

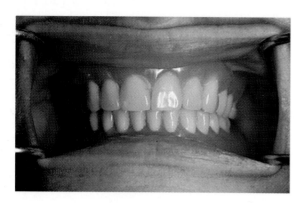

Figure 10-43

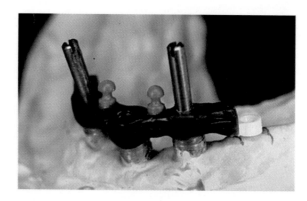

Figure 10-44

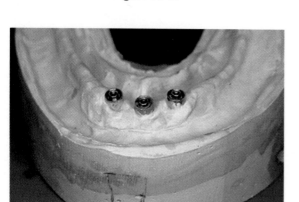

Figure 10-45

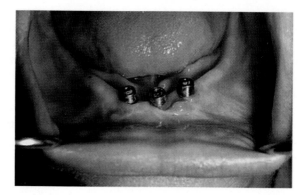

Figure 10-46

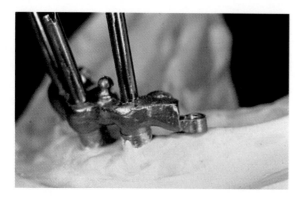

Figure 10-47

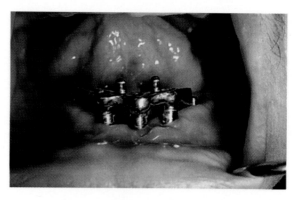

Figure 10-48

fashion. Castings are reclaimed and reverified to the master cast.

The framework fit is verified passively and secured with gold screws. The interfaces between the gold cylinders and the abutments are examined for accuracy of fit. If any discrepancies are noted the bar is cut, soldering indexes are made, and the framework is returned to the laboratory for soldering. If no changes are to be made to the framework, it is returned to the laboratory for final polishing and processing of the overdentures.

Overdentures are processed using recommended manufacturer's directions for processing stud attachments.

CEKA ATTACHMENTS WITH SECONDARY FRAMEWORK PROCESSED INSIDE

Ceka attachments have been used in dentistry for precision removable partial dentures for decades. The attachment male is adjustable for customizing retention. A secondary framework is cast to retain the male attachment. The worn attachments can be replaced easily by unscrewing.

The patient in Fig. 10-50 had desired a fixed prosthesis originally. Onlay grafting was completed with placement of seven implants. The patient was a known smoker and convinced the surgeon that she had quit smoking before the onlay graft was contemplated. She was also advised to wear her treatment denture after graft replacement for cosmetics only. A soft diet was recommended, and the denture was to be left out at night. The patient was noncompliant with the surgeon's wishes, and multiple implants were lost. Stress in the patient's life contributed to her starting to smoke again after grafting procedures. She also admitted to wearing the denture 24 hours per day and to chewing as well. The four remaining implants were used to fabricate an overdenture. An attachment bar was cast after a trial denture setup was completed (Fig. 10-51). The trial setup is necessary to determine if adequate intermaxillary space exists for the attachment bar and secondary frame without violating freeway space.

The attachment bar was made incorporating receptacles for six female components (Figs. 10-52 to 10-55). Only three attachments were used initially. Another framework was made to be processed into the overdenture while retaining the male attachments (see Fig. 10-53). Full palatal coverage was used for the first year (see Fig. 10-54). The palate was removed, and additional attachments were added after 1 year of function (Fig. 10-56). Inadequate tissue contours even after grafting precluded fabricating a fixed prosthesis. An overdenture was required to restore facial contour while allowing access for hygiene (Figs. 10-57 to 10-61). Successful

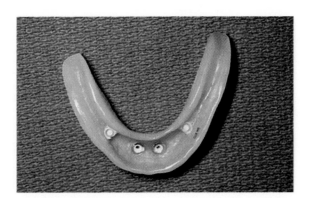

Figure 10-49

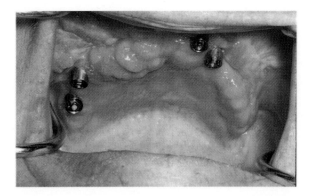

Figure 10-50

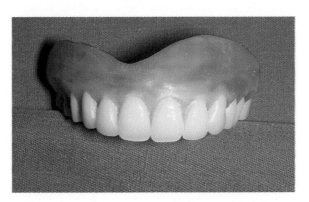

Figure 10-51

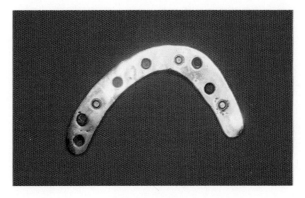

Figure 10-52

treatment with bone grafting is dependent on many factors, especially patient compliance.

UNCONNECTED FIXTURES

Many attachments have been manufactured for fabricating implant-retained overdentures without using an attachment bar. The attachments are designed to connect directly to the abutment. There are fewer components and less clinical and laboratory time used; therefore fees are lower, making this an economic alternative to an attachment bar-retained overdenture. Impressions, try-ins, records, and procedures are identical, except that bar fabrication is eliminated. A processed acrylic base allows for a more secure clinical record making.

MAGNETIC ATTACHMENTS

The development of rare-earth element magnets has greatly increased the magnetic force available for prosthetic retention in a clinically applicable size. Magnetic systems incorporate the magnet, which is either a neodymium-iron-boron alloy or a samarium cobalt alloy. Both alloys corrode quickly in oral fluids and must be encased in a protective coating to pre-

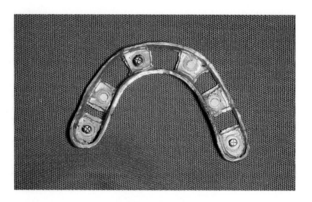

Figure 10-53

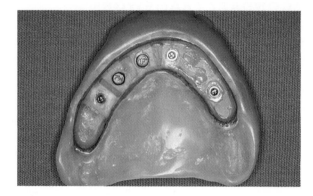

Figure 10-54

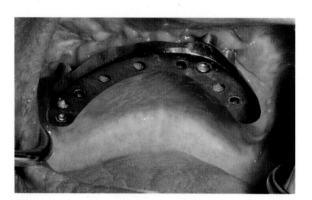

Figure 10-55

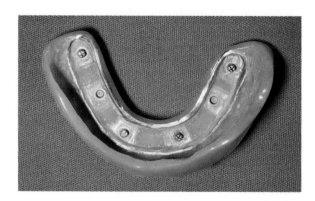

Figure 10-56

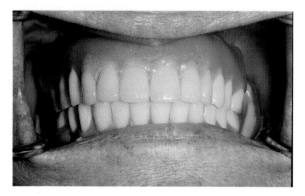

Figure 10-57

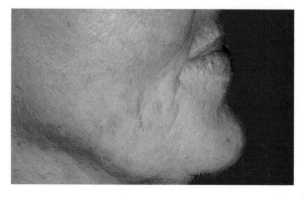

Figure 10-58

vent contamination and loss of magnetism. The second part of the magnet system is the ferromagnetic keeper (Figs. 10-62 and 10-63). This component is designed to screw onto the abutment and is made of a ferromagnetic alloy. The magnet is retained in the denture.

The magnets experienced loss of magnetism when exposed to the heat of processing; therefore a plastic magnet analogue (if available) must be used until processing has been completed. The magnets can be picked up with auto-polymerizing resin at the delivery appointment (Figs. 10-64

to 10-66). The Shriner magnet system has a series of laboratory analogues that allow processed base fabrications, as well as processing with magnet analogues (Fig. 10-67). The magnet analogues are unscrewed, and the plastic-encased magnets are screwed in at the delivery appointment.

Magnetic systems have shown problems involving corrosion (as previously mentioned). Even with a metal or a plastic encasement, the forces of mastication can wear through the encasement. Corrosion and rapid loss of magnetism occur once the encasement is broken.

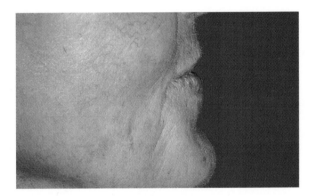

Figure 10-59

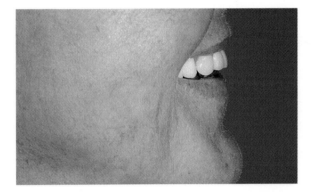

Figure 10-60

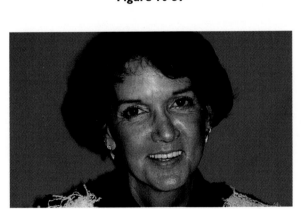

Figure 10-61

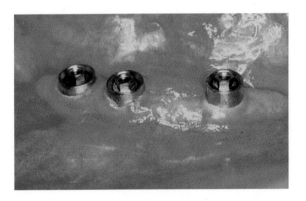

Figure 10-62

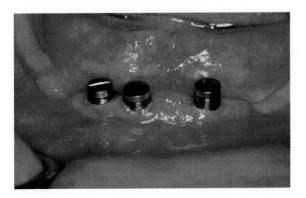

Figure 10-63

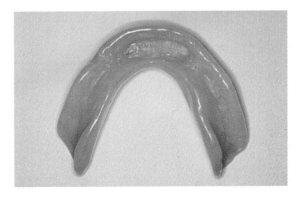

Figure 10-64

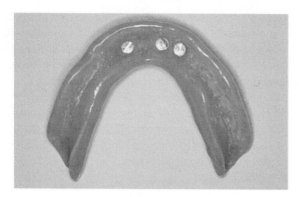

Figure 10-65

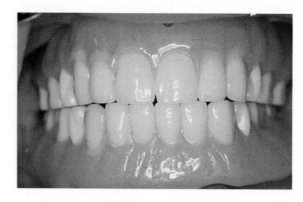

Figure 10-66

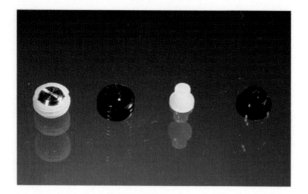

Figure 10-67

CHAPTER 11

Osseointegrated Implants in Combination with Vascularized Bone Grafts: Surgical and Prosthodontic Considerations

Jeffrey E. Rubenstein
Neal D. Futran
Philip Worthington

SURGICAL CONSIDERATIONS

Reconstruction of the mandible and maxilla makes frequent use today of free vascularized tissue transfer.[1] This enables the surgeon skilled in microvascular techniques to repair very extensive defects arising from cancer ablation, congenital anomalies, or trauma. It is important that the implant surgeon and the prosthodontist understand the essentials of free vascularized grafts and the impact of this relatively recent technology on oral rehabilitation. Much has changed since microvascular reconstruction of the mandible was first described by Strauch and colleagues in 1971.[2] Twenty years later, Urken and colleagues[3] reported a series of 71 cases of mandibular reconstruction using microvascular free flaps, with a success rate of 94%. Fifteen of those patients had endosseous implants placed at the time of the graft and subsequently wore implant-supported prostheses.

The most obvious advantage of the free vascularized bone graft compared with the conventional nonvascularized autogenous graft is that the transferred tissue has its own blood supply from the beginning. It does not have to "gain" a blood supply from its immediate new surroundings, which in so many cancer patients has severely impaired vitality as a result of surgery and/or irradiation. In addition, vascularized bone primarily heals to native bone, as in a fracture, and may sustain loading earlier than a nonvascularized graft.

Not all mandibular or maxillary resection defects demand reconstruction, but some have such devastating effects on function and appearance that it is essential. A prime example is the major defect in the symphyseal region, where reconstruction is necessary and inherently difficult and where the free vascularized bone graft is the optimal method of repair. By contrast, in the posterior mandible the vascularized bone has no overwhelming superiority, and in some cases reconstruction may not be essential unless the patient wishes to have a functional dental restoration.

The aims of mandibular reconstruction are to restore the three-dimensional shape of the jaw, to restore the contours of the lower face while maintaining tongue mobility and ultimately providing dental prostheses with an acceptable occlusion, and to provide oral continence.

For maxillary defects the goals for reconstruction include the elimination of a communication between the mouth and the nasal and/or sinus cavities, the creation of a bony archi-

tecture that establishes a base of support for implant placement, and ultimately the replacement of the missing dentition. This effort should facilitate and not compromise speech and swallowing and provide a restoration of normal anatomic contours of the midface. Free vascularized tissue is necessary when the existing structures do not provide enough support, stability, and retention for a prosthesis.

Factors to consider in planning the reconstruction include the site and size of the defect; the associated soft-tissue deficiency; and the involvement of the skin, muscles, nerves, and vessels. Furthermore, the patient may have already been irradiated or may need radiation postoperatively. In planning the procedure, the surgeon will consider the patient's age and prognosis, general health, diet and activity level, motivation, and the family dynamics. Specific indications for reconstruction using free vascularized grafts include the following:

1. Full-thickness defects (involving the mucosa, bone, and skin)
2. Failure of previous attempts at reconstruction
3. Severe osteoradionecrosis
4. Loss of tooth-bearing segments necessary for functional dental restoration

Flap Selection and Operative Procedure

Many types of free flaps have been designed and used for jaw reconstruction. Those noted here are the ones most commonly used for mandibular and, more recently, maxillary reconstruction.

Fibula free flap. Because the donor site is remote from the recipient site, two surgical teams can work simultaneously, one harvesting the composite graft from the leg and the other resecting the jaw.[4,5] This shortens the total operative time for the patient. The fibula has been shown to be suitable for the installation of osseointegrated implants. In the adult male a length of bone up to 25 cm may be harvested, based on the peroneal vessels and accompanied by a paddle of skin and some of the soleus muscle (Fig. 11-1). The straight fibula can be subjected (with care) to multiple wedge osteotomies to make the bone conform to the curve of the mandible or maxilla. Freedom to rotate the skin paddle relative to the bone is limited. The bone is mainly cortical, and the effective height is commonly about 1 cm. Before choosing this flap, the blood supply to the leg is investigated using color-flow Doppler ultrasonography, which also helps to identify the cutaneous perforating vessels. Surprisingly the morbidity at the donor site is low. In many cases primary skin closure can be achieved; the leg is splinted for about 4 days, and then ambulation begins.

Iliac crest flap. The iliac crest flap is based on the deep circumflex iliac vessels and provides a greater quantity of cancellous bone and a greater height of bone than any other site (up to 2½ cm)[5] (Fig. 11-2). The two-team approach is feasible. The graft comes with a skin paddle and/or a muscle paddle from the internal oblique muscle. This flap is useful for through-and-through defects (the skin being inset into the external defect and the muscle being inset into the oral mucosa). Because this flap tends to be very bulky, considerable soft-tissue thinning and recontouring may be needed. At the donor site, repair must be meticulous because of the risk of hernia. Gait is disturbed for 3 to 4 weeks, and physical therapy aids recovery.

Scapula flap. The scapula flap is based on the deep circumflex scapular vessels and provides a somewhat limited volume of bone from the lateral border of the scapula[6] (Fig. 11-3). The associated skin paddle can be positioned freely relative to the bone. With this flap the two-team approach is not feasible. The flap may be appropriate for small osseous defects associated with complicated soft-tissue defects, especially in the midface region.

Radial forearm flap. The radial forearm flap provides a skin paddle of thin, pliable soft tissue that may be innervated by the antebrachial cutaneous nerve. At the donor site the scar is often unsightly. Bone is seldom included because it is limited in volume and vertical height, therefore making it a poor candidate for implant placement. Furthermore, there is a risk of fracture of the radius. A 6-week period of immobilization is necessary after harvest of the graft.

Operative procedure. For microvascular bone grafting the usual sequence of events is as follows:

1. If the tumor has not penetrated the mandibular buccal bone cortex, a reconstruction plate is adapted to the bone with at least three screw holes on either side of the resection area. The plate and screws are then removed.
2. The tumor excision is completed, and the recipient vessels are identified.
3. The plate is then reapplied and screwed into place.
4. The graft is harvested, osteotomized as needed, and adapted to the plate and the gap.
5. Water-tight mucosal closure without tension is achieved intraorally.
6. Microvascular anastomoses are completed, and viability is assessed. Usually up to 4 hours of warm ischemia time can be tolerated.

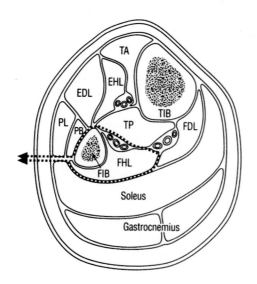

TA	Tibialis Anterior	TP	Tibialis Posterior
EHL	Extensor Hallucis Longus	FDL	Flexor Digitorum Longus
EDL	Extensor Digitorum Longus	FHL	Flexor Hallucis Longus
PL	Peroneus Longus	TIB	Tibia
PB	Peroneus Brevis	FIB	Fibula

Figure 11-1

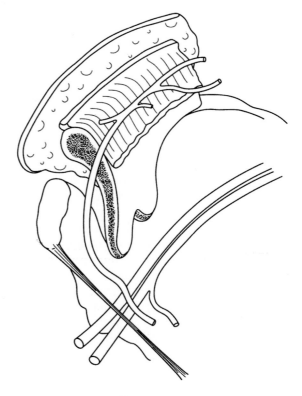

Figure 11-2

Where the tumor has penetrated the buccal bone cortex, the reconstruction plate cannot be adapted before tumor extirpation. Under these circumstances one may use pin fixation of the retained fragments with the condyles in the fossae, or a universal reconstruction plate may be used to achieve the same goal.

For congenital anomalies and trauma cases, a similar treatment sequence is followed but modified to accommodate individual variation and anatomic requirements that obviously vary from those of tumor ablation surgery. Bone placement may be matched to the mandibular alveolus. Trauma may differ in that the initial plating of the fractured segments needs to precede introduction of the free-tissue transfer. The maxillary cases often present difficulty in obtaining a base of bone on which to secure the grafts. Secure fixation is ideally achieved at the anterior maxillary and zygomatic buttress regions.

Timing of Implant Placement

Implants may be placed into the bone graft at the time of tissue transfer so patient can enjoy an earlier return to function.[7] After a period of 4 to 6 months for osseointegration to develop, the implants can be uncovered, the abutments can be connected, and a prosthesis can be constructed. Some clinicians feel that it is difficult to achieve ideal placement of the implants under these circumstances and prefer to place the implants at a secondary stage. Since the soft tissues so frequently need thinning and adjusting, that may be done at the same time.

Primary versus Secondary Reconstruction

If bony reconstruction can be done at the time of tumor excision, the patient benefits psychologically and returns to function earlier. This may be particularly important in cases where the neoplasm is advanced and the prognosis is poor, because early palliation and improvement in the quality of life is a priority. Furthermore, one major operative procedure is always preferred. When the jaw reconstruction is done as a secondary procedure, the patient will frequently have undergone radiation therapy in the interval. The development of scarring during the interval may cause residual parts of the mandible to drift out of position, and correcting this misalignment is sometimes difficult. The resultant ischemia and fibrosis make the later surgery more difficult; this applies also to placement of the vascularized tissue transfer. Success in vascularized tissue transfer depends on precise surgery, careful postoperative monitoring, and a true team effort with early involvement of the nursing staff, speech therapist, and others.

Vascularized Bone Grafts as Recipient Sites for Endosseous Implants

When placing implants into vascularized bone grafts, the same meticulous technique must be used as in any other circumstance. The vertical height of the available bone is often limited, which means that it is advantageous to strive for bicortical anchorage whenever possible. The ratio between the height of the superstructure and the height of the endosseous implant—the S/I ratio (superstructure/implant ratio)—is of great significance from a biomechanical point of view (Fig. 11-4). Therefore if the free vascularized bone graft (such as a fibula) is aligned with the lower border of the remaining mandible, the S/I ratio may well be unfavorable (Fig. 11-5). By deliberately misaligning the fibula section, moving it in an occlusal direction by 1/2 to 1 cm, this factor

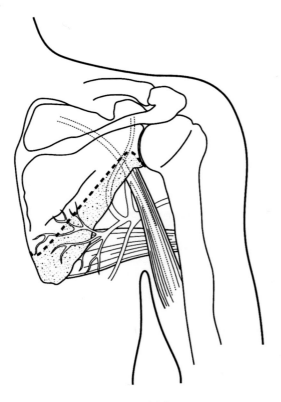

Figure 11-3

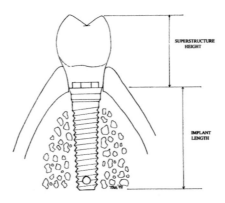

Figure 11-4

may be much improved. The discrepancy at the lower border is unlikely to be detectable since the soft tissue that accompanies the graft successfully disguises the misalignment (Fig. 11-6).

The soft tissue that surrounds the future abutments is frequently found to be too thick and the tissue too mobile to be satisfactory as peri-implant material. Years of experience have shown that mobile tissue around implants can result in a hyperplastic response unless the oral hygiene is impeccable. Therefore it is often desirable to thin the peri-implant tissue—sometimes repeatedly—until the tissue is thin and tethered to the bone.

In summary it may be said that the development of free vascularized tissue transfer has been a major advance in cancer reconstructive surgery. It is important that all members of the teams involved—ablationists, microvascular surgeon, and implant team—should understand the nature and the problems of each other's work so that their combined efforts may yield the maximal benefit for the patient. From a practical point of view it is advantageous that a complete treatment plan be developed at the beginning, including plans for oral rehabilitation with implant-supported prostheses. This plan should be submitted in its entirety to insurance carriers so that one may avoid the unfortunate situation where a patient is granted coverage for the resection and bony reconstruction but is later denied coverage for the implant surgery and special prosthodontic care that is so necessary.

PROSTHODONTIC CONSIDERATIONS

With the introduction of the aforementioned surgical reconstruction procedures, a new era has dawned for rehabilitation of patients who have defects of the maxilla and/or mandible secondary to congenital anomalies, trauma, or tumor ablation surgery and postoperative radiotherapy to eradicate carcinomas of the head and neck. In the past, lateral defects of the mandible were not commonly restored to establish continuity of the mandible. For anterior defects of the mandible, various approaches using alloplastic materials,

titanium, or Vitallium trays generally proved ineffective because of difficulty in maintaining tissue coverage. For unilateral or anterior maxillary defects in partially dentate patients, obturators have proven to be effective rehabilitation. However, for edentulous patients or patients who have had bilateral total maxillectomies, prosthodontic rehabilitation often is much less satisfactory from the standpoint of providing a prosthesis that has appropriate support, stability, and retention necessary to meet the functional requirements for such patients.

With the advent and application of both nonvascularized and microvascular free-flap reconstruction of both mandibular and maxillary surgically created defects and the placement of osseointegrated implants, meaningful rehabilitation previously only dreamed of is now routinely accomplished. However, given the fact that these surgical procedures are relatively new, much still needs to be learned and implemented to improve the functional and cosmetic results.[7] The following section addresses these concerns and recommends solutions based on clinical experience gained thus far.

MANDIBULAR REHABILITATION
Posterior Lateral Defects

For the patient who has the body (or body, ramus, and condyle) resected, restored mandibular continuity is essential to restore normal function (Figs. 11-7 and 11-8). Either nonvascularized iliac crest grafts or vascularized ilium, fibula, or to a lesser extent scapula have been used to accomplish this goal (Fig. 11-9). Several considerations must be taken into account to adequately provide implant rehabilitation for these grafted cases.[8,9] These variables differ for the patient who has not undergone mandibular reconstruction and include the following:

1. Tongue tethering
2. Maintenance of arch form
3. Oral competency
4. Vertical dimension of occlusion
5. Superstructure/ implant ratio
6. Interabutment/intraabutment tissue quality

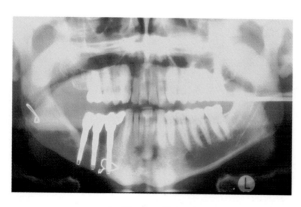

Figure 11-5

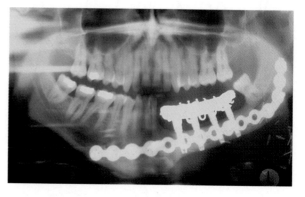

Figure 11-6

All of these compromises have been shown to present significant challenges to satisfactory rehabilitation.

Tongue tethering secondary to reconstructive efforts can result in a limited and/or aberrant range of motion of the tongue, which results in compromises in speech, swallowing, and mastication (Fig. 11-10). Furthermore, there may be sensory and/or motor deficits resulting from tumor resection. The lingual contours of the prosthesis frequently need to be modified so the tongue can function in a way that is compatible with the prosthesis rather than antagonistic to it. Depending on the site of the primary tumor, tongue tethering can present posterior-laterally or anteriorly. Regardless of the tethering location, this phenomenon impacts negatively in the making of impressions of the reconstructed arch and implant positions. The limited range of motion of the tongue can compromise its ability to direct the bolus of food onto the occlusal surfaces of the teeth, thereby compromising the patient's ability to effectively masticate. Frequently this compromise necessitates reduction of the vertical dimension of occlusion to coordinate with the tongue's range of motion. Speech compromise can result from tethering of the tongue, which can also necessitate altered contours of the prosthesis to improve speech. Assessment of this concern with a well-trained speech pathologist is invaluable in providing assistance to the patient to maximize his or her speech potential.

Maintenance of the arch form is critical for the overall rehabilitation effort. Plating or use of external pin fixation of the mandible before resection to maintain the relationship of the segments before grafting is essential. In cases where this has not been accomplished, the distribution of the implants has been unfavorable and necessitates compromises in the design of the implant framework and altered contours of the prosthesis, and it often results in compromises in lip support and tongue posture (Fig. 11-11).

Vertical dimension of occlusion is a much more challenging issue with patients who have undergone graft reconstruction of the mandible. One practical consideration is that these patients typically are not able to wear conventional prostheses after reconstruction. The prolonged healing intervals after grafting and subsequent implant placement and phase two surgery often leave the muscles of mastication and resultant jaw posture essentially nonfunctional relative to occlusal contact, often for a period of a year or more while rehabilitation is being pursued. Assessment of vertical dimension of occlusion in this type of patient is very different than for a patient who is having immediate or conventional dentures fabricated. An estimate needs to be made, and typically one should err on the side of a reduced versus an increased vertical dimension of occlusion relative to the design of the prosthesis. Furthermore, it is not uncommon in mandibular

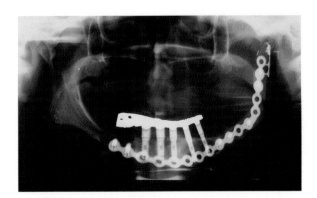

Figure 11-7

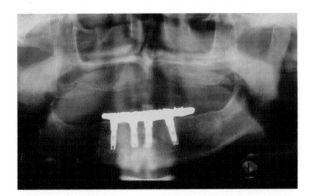

Figure 11-8

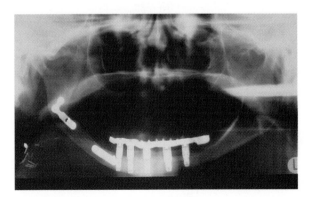

Figure 11-9

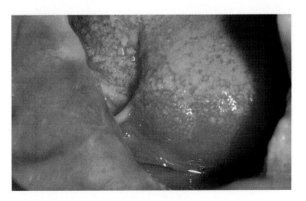

Figure 11-10

bone graft reconstruction patients, particularly those who have had radiotherapy, to be dealing with restriction of oral opening. Not only does this compromise the vertical dimension of occlusion, but it also limits access to the oral cavity for placing components such as impression copings, trays, and so on (Fig. 11-12, *A* and *B*). Implant surgery is often performed for patients under general anesthesia, during which time the patient is asleep and paralyzed, creating a very different environment relative to oral opening when compared with the patient being awake and the muscles of mastication fully active. Therefore clinical prosthodontic procedures generally have more limited oral access when compared with the patient's surgical management.

Oral competency also factors into this patient population as a complication that affects the prosthesis design. For patients who have lost motor function and/or sensation to the lip secondary to resection and reconstruction, control of saliva and the food bolus becomes significantly more challenging (Fig. 11-13). Developing the contours of the prosthesis that appropriately support the lip, assist in allowing the patient to achieve oral valving, and do not contribute to lip biting are often difficult to accomplish. As previously stated the vertical dimension of occlusion directly affects whether the patient can successfully achieve oral competency. A prosthetic design that does not provide the patient with the potential for achieving oral competency is a failure despite pro-

viding the patient with improved masticatory function and esthetics.

Soft-tissue management around and between abutments is another critical factor in achieving success with implant rehabilitation of the graft reconstruction patient. More often than not, the oral topography after grafting results in altered anatomy that is devoid of a gingivobuccal or lingual sulcus as well as provision for a zone of attached tissue in the region where transmucosal abutments come through the graft. Tissue movement about the abutments during normal oral function results in nonattached tissues becoming irritated and inflamed (Fig. 11-14). This, combined with the patient having more difficulty maintaining a plaque free environment around these abutments, can result in an unfavorable tissue response. Successful implant prosthodontic treatment is entirely dependent on maintenance of tissue health to ensure long-term service.

Graft placement to align the graft with the inferior border of the mandible often results in an unfavorable S/I ratio. Secondary grafting to onlay a graft to increase its vertical height has been attempted but unfortunately rarely results in restoration of the original height of the jaw. At present, the S/I ratio does not seem to have any bearing on the conventional dogma related to the crown/root ratio for natural teeth. Although a crown/root ratio of a least 1:1 is considered ideal, it is not uncommon for the S/I ratio in graft reconstruction

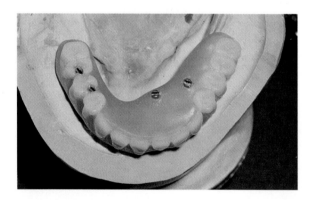

Figure 11-11

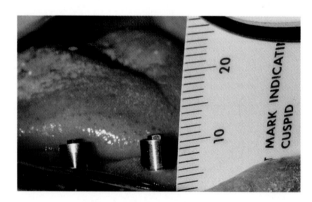

Figure 11-12, A

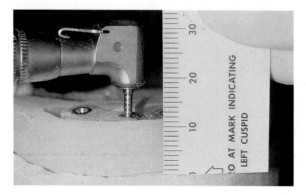

Figure 11-12, B

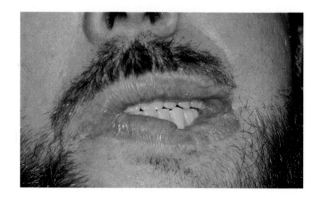

Figure 11-13

patients to exceed 3:1 (Figs. 11-5 and 11-15). The replacement of missing teeth and supporting structures necessitated in these cases has been accomplished with a variety of prosthetic designs and materials. A conventional hybrid design is one option, using acrylic teeth processed to a framework with gingival shade resin. Porcelain fused to metal can also be used with either gingival shade resin veneer or gingival shade porcelain (Figs. 11-16 and 11-17). If hygiene access is compromised, an overdenture-type design can be considered to allow for removal of the dental portion of the prosthesis, which provides access to the abutments and the supporting bar or free-standing implant overdenture retainers on indi-

vidual abutments (Fig. 11-18, *A* and *B*). Longer follow-up is needed to determine what an acceptable ratio should be as a treatment goal. Patients thus far treated with what are thought to be unfavorable S/I ratios have not as yet experienced implant loss, prosthesis failure, or other complications.

The edentulous patient who has had tumor resection and graft reconstruction generally is not a candidate for successful function with a conventional tissue-supported prosthesis. Although some centers have advocated the use of implant overdentures as the treatment of choice, it is the experience of the authors that a nonremovable implant-supported prosthesis is preferable when possible. In particular, the patient

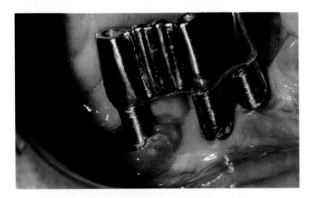

Figure 11-14

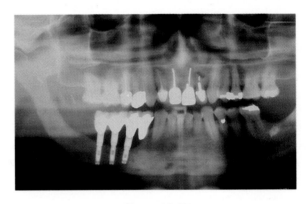

Figure 11-15

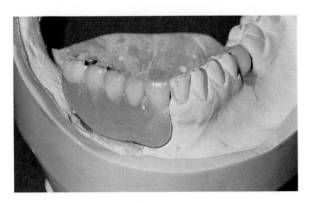

Figure 11-16

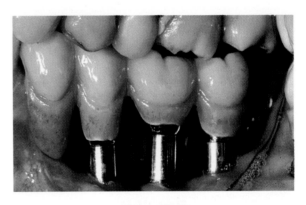

Figure 11-17

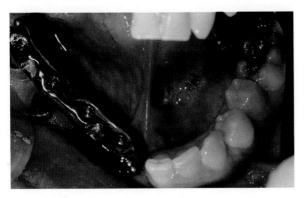

Figure 11-18, A

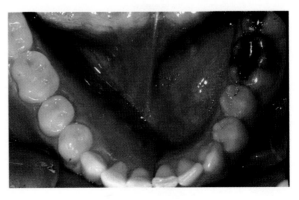

Figure 11-18, B

who has had both surgery and radiation treatment seems to benefit most by not having the prosthesis supported by the soft tissues. To date our center has enjoyed a high level of success with edentulous patients who have had surgical resection/graft reconstruction, implants placed secondarily, and restoration with implant-supported prostheses. Similarly, patients who have had surgical resection/graft reconstruction, postoperative radiation, implant placement with preplacemnt and postplacement hyperbaric oxygen treatment (i.e., the Marx protocol[11]), and an implant-supported prostheses have also experienced a high level of success (Figs. 11-7, 11-8, 11-19, and 11-20). In fact, over a period of more than 10 years, the authors have not experienced implant loss in any patient who has had radiation treatment, hyperbaric oxygen, and implants placed in the anterior mandible. The results of these consecutively treated patients are currently being prepared for publication.

Anterior Arch Reconstruction

Patients having the anterior arch of the mandible reconstructed have been treated with a nonremovable implant-supported prostheses. As previously stated, the quality of the soft tissue around the abutments and the sulcus depth, such that access for oral hygiene procedures can be accomplished, are critical for long-term success (Fig 11-21, A and B).

Partially Edentulous Reconstruction

For partially edentulous patients, graft placement typically results in an unfavorable S/I ratio and a lack of attached tissue about the implant abutments. Although neither of these concerns has been insurmountable, it is too early to determine their effects on long-term survival of these rehabilitative efforts.

Electrolysis is often necessary to eliminate hair growth of fibula microvascular flaps (Fig. 11-22, A and B). A variety of designs for prosthodontic rehabilitation, both fixed and removable, have been employed for partially edentulous patients. The chief concern for the partially edentulous patient is the replacement of not only the missing teeth but also of the supporting structures. In this regard it is critical that access for abutment hygiene be given strong consideration in the prosthesis design. Soft-tissue complications secondary to a lack of attached tissue have been proven to be a significant management problem.

MAXILLARY RECONSTRUCTION

Use of various bone grafts to restore continuity to the mandible has led to a natural extension of these techniques for maxillary defects. Although partially edentulous patients have functioned successfully with obturator prostheses, a trend toward closure of oral/antral and/or sinus communi-

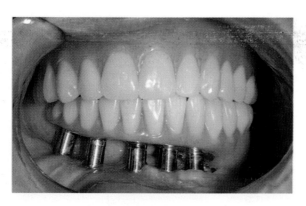

Figure 11-19

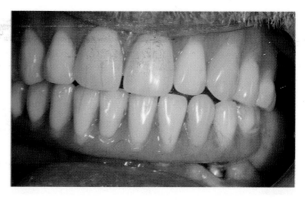

Figure 11-20

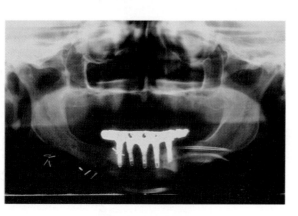

Figure 11-21, A

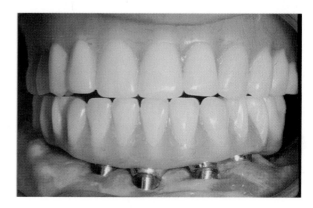

Figure 11-21, B

cations is currently being pursued to eliminate the need for a removable obturator prosthesis. In its place are attempts to provide an adequate volume of bone and soft tissue to provide a base into which implants can be placed and ultimate missing dentition restored. This more recent application of implant rehabilitation at our center has proven to be even more challenging from a surgical implant placement and prosthodontic perspective. Although there is some overlap regarding concerns for surgical reconstruction/implant prosthodontic rehabilitation of the maxilla as compared with the mandible, there are also other factors that are unique to maxillary rehabilitative efforts that are elucidated in this section.

Bilateral total maxillectomy perhaps is the ultimate rehabilitation challenge. In the past, rehabilitation efforts of unreconstructed defects were more an exercise in futility rather than meaningfully restoring the patient to normal oral function. Perhaps the ability to surgically reconstruct an entire maxilla results in the most dramatic rehabilitation currently available to date in the head and neck region. Grafting, implant placement, and fabrication of an implant-supported prosthesis that restores speech, swallowing, mastication, and deglutition to a patient with no potential for normal oral function is indeed dramatic. In the few cases treated thus far the authors have experienced prosthodontic designs that have

required the development of anterior and buccal cantilevers that exceed conventional dogma for maxillary implant rehabilitation for those edentulous patients restored with maxillary implant-supported prostheses. Although it is generally recommended that posterior cantilevers do not exceed 10 mm for maxillary implant prostheses,[12] no specific recommendations relative to anterior cantilevering have been reported. One such example of a prosthetic design necessitated an anterior cantilever of 20 mm (Fig. 11-23, *A*) to allow for appropriate anterior tooth position and a buccal cantilever of 10 mm (Fig. 11-23, *B*) on the left that would be compatible with the arch form and tooth position of the existing mandibular teeth. This design was dictated by implant placement in a maxilla reconstructed with a vascularized fibula graft after bilateral total maxillectomy where the arch form was foreshortened and posterior to the original preresection configuration. To allow for appropriate tooth position and lip support, the implant-supported prosthesis was designed so that it would accommodate the arch form and tooth position of the patient's existing mandibular teeth (Fig. 11-24, *A* to *C*). Similarly, Fig. 11-25, *A* and *B* demonstrates the same situation for a patient whose maxilla was reconstructed with a scapula vascularized graft.

Although it is not uncommon for implant surgeons to be criticized for less than optimal implant placement despite

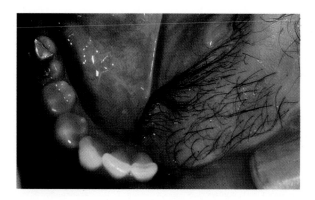

Figure 11-22, A

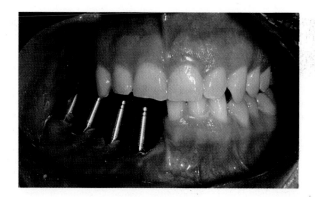

Figure 11-22, B

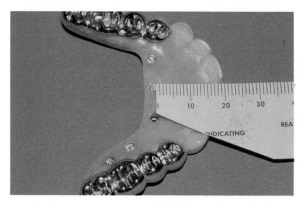

Figure 11-23, A

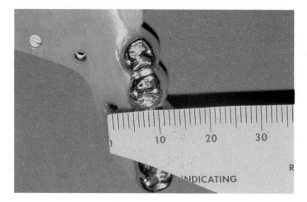

Figure 11-23, B

being provided surgical templates to assist in this decision-making process, the reconstructed maxilla apparently puts this concern in an entirely new realm. Furthermore, it is not known what the long-term prospects for continued osseointegration are for these excessively long anterior cantilevers for implants placed in grafted reconstructed maxillas.

Provisional restorations converted from preimplant placement tissue-borne prostheses (generally used to accomplish surgical stent fabrication) are developed by indexing temporary cylinders (polymer) into the treatment prosthesis and then cutting back to the anticipated contours of the

implant-supported prosthesis that is being planned for long-term use. These provisional restorations have served a variety of functions:

1. Provide provisional (progressive) loading to the implants and bone graft.
2. Allow the patient to assess the prosthetic design.
3. See what difficulties might result relative to oral hygiene access.
4. Test the contours of the prosthesis relative to facilitating speech and swallowing.
5. Assist in determining appropriate lip support and vertical dimension of occlusion.

Generally speaking, the greater the anatomic compromise, the greater the need for a provisional restoration to assist in the assessment and ultimate design of the long-term treatment. Furthermore, provisional restorations provide for earlier rehabilitation of the patient and also provide for a spare prosthesis once treatment is completed.

SUMMARY
Patients with significant compromise to their oral anatomy associated with loss resulting from trauma, cancer ablation surgery, or maldevelopment of the jaws are now able to be

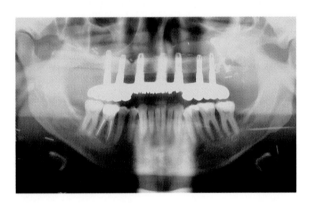

Figure 11-24, A

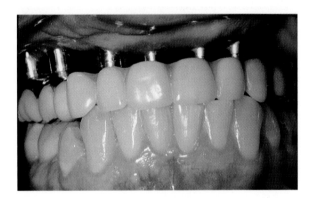

Figure 11-24, B

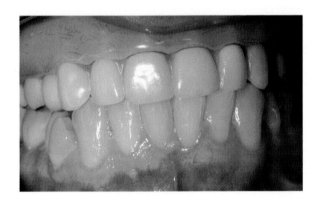

Figure 11-24, C

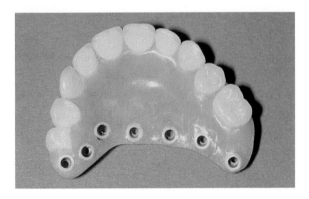

Figure 11-25, A

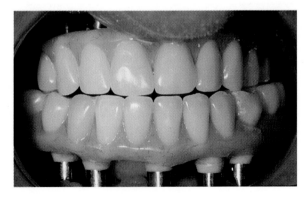

Figure 11-25, B

rehabilitated using vascularized grafts that import bone and soft tissue to the oral cavity to restore these compromises of the oral anatomy. With these grafts as a base for rehabilitation, dental implants can be placed and used as a support system for replacing missing dentition and associated structures. Although these new techniques are in their infancy, further refinements will certainly continue to enhance these rehabilitation efforts. Patients with severely compromised oral anatomy can be provided with vastly improved oral function.

References

1. Turk JB, Vuillemin T, Raveh J: Revascularized bone grafts for craniofacial reconstruction, *Otolaryngol Clin North Am* 27:955, 1994.
2. Strauch B, Bloomberg AE, Lewin ML: An experimental approach to mandibular replacement: island vascular composite rib grafts, *Brit J Plast Reconstr Surg* 24:334, 1971.
3. Urken ML, Weinberg H, Vickery C et al: Oromandibular reconstruction using microvascular composite free flaps: report of 71 cases and a new classification scheme for bony, soft tissue and neurological defects, *Arch Otolaryngol Head Neck Surg* 117:733, 1991.
4. Wolff KD, Ervens J, Herzog K et al: Experience with the osteocutaneous fibula flap: an analysis of 24 consecutive reconstructions of composite mandibular defects, *J Craniomaxillofac Surg* 24:330, 1996.
5. Haughey BH, Fredrickson JM, Lerrick AJ et al: Fibular and iliac crest osteomuscular free flap reconstruction of the oral cavity, *Laryngoscope* 104:1305, 1994.
6. Vinzenz KG, Holle J, Wuringer E et al: Prefabrication of combined scapula flaps for microsurgical reonstruction in oromaxillofacial defects: a new method, *J Craniomaxillofac Surg* 24:214, 1996.
7. Sclaaroff A, Haughey B, Gay WD et al: Immediate mandibular reconstruction and placement of dnetal implants at the time of ablative surgery, *Oral Path Oral Surg Oral Med* 78:711, 1994.
8. Esser E, Wagner W: Dental implants following radical oral cancer surgery and adjuvant radiotherapy, *Int J Oral Maxillofac Implants* 12:552, 1997.
9. Aldegheri A, Beloni D, Blanc JL et al: Dental rehabilitaion using osseointegrated implants: treatment of oro-maxillo-facial cancer: a preliminary study of 7 cases, *Rev Stomatol Chir Maxillofac* 97:108, 1996.
10. Schmelzeisen R, Ptok M, Schonweiler R et al: Reconstruction of speech and chewing function after extensive tumor resection in the area of the jaw and face, *Laryngorhinootologie* 75:231, 1996.
11. Marx RE: A new concept in the treatment of osteoradionecrosis, *J Oral Maxillofac Surg* 41:351, 1983.
12. Branemark P-I, Zarb GA, Albrektsson T: *Tissue integrated prostheses: osseointegration in clinical dentistry*, Chicago, 1985, Quintessence.

Special Cases

The patients presented in this chapter have implant-supported prostheses restoring a variety of congenital and acquired defects. The prosthetic and laboratory techniques are beyond the scope of this text but are shown as further examples of implant applications.

BONE GRAFTING—ONCOLOGIC DEFECTS

The patient in Figs. 12-1 and 12-2 had resections for ameloblastoma at ages 3 weeks and 6 months. Treatment partials were worn by the patient until the age of 18 years. Radiographs of the anatomic defect can be seen in Figs. 12-3 and 12-4. Bone was harvested from the iliac crest and grafted onto the maxillary defect. These implants were placed in the

graft (Figs. 12-5 and 12-6). The finished prosthesis is seen in Figs. 12-6 to 12-11.

MANDIBULAR SPLIT-FRAME PROSTHESIS

The patient shown in Figs. 12-12 to 12-16 had implants angled such that the screw access holes interfered with the strength and esthetics of the incisal edges of the anterior teeth. She also had a hysterical reaction to the display of 2 to 3 mm of abutment, which was only visible during photography with the maximum retraction of the lower lip. A split-frame prosthesis was designed to provide a superstructure that compensated for implant angulation and provided coverage of the abutments down to the mucosa. This design was

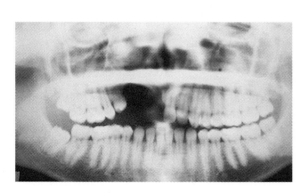

Figure 12-1

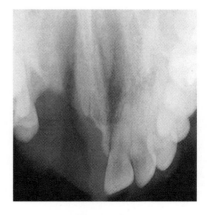

Figure 12-2

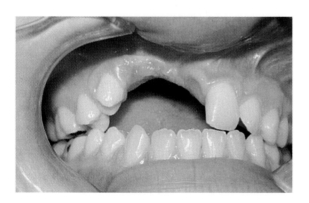

Figure 12-3

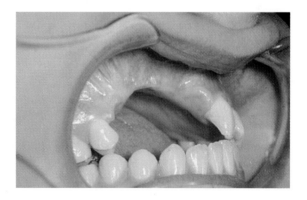

Figure 12-4

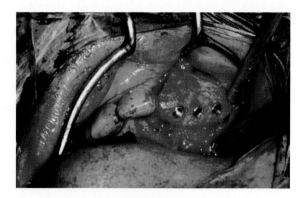

Figure 12-5

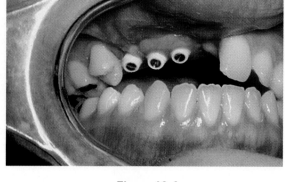

Figure 12-6

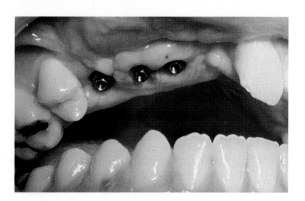

Figure 12-7

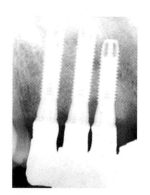

Figure 12-8

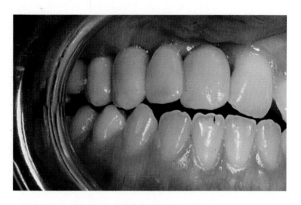

Figure 12-9

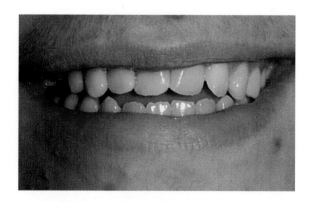

Figure 12-10

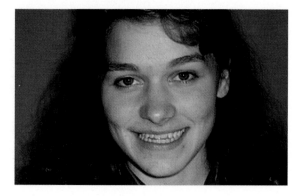

Figure 12-11

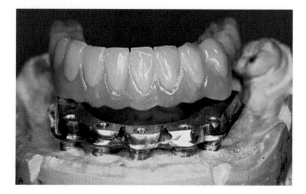

Figure 12-12

first presented by Patrick Henry, DDS (Perth, Australia). Dovetail attachments (PD) were placed horizontally parallel to one another in the inferior screw-retained segment. The veneered superior framework was retained with set screws.

ACQUIRED AND CONGENITAL DEFECTS

Cleft palate patients and patients who have had surgical resections for tumor removal may have anatomic defects that require prosthetic replacement. Traditional prosthetics necessitate the use of existing teeth or other anatomy for retaining

the prosthesis. The lack of retention for prosthetics often leaves the patient severely compromised functionally. Implant placement provides much greater retention for prosthetics, improving speech and other functions (Fig. 12-17).

MAXILLECTOMY DEFECTS

The patient in Fig. 12-18 has a left maxillectomy to remove a squamous cell carcinoma. She had worn an edentulous obturator for 20 years with little success. Her speech was hypernasal. Food and liquids leaked out of her nose during deglutition. Three implants were placed in the remaining

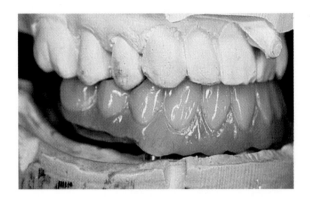

Figure 12-13

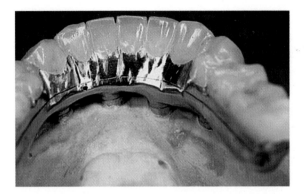

Figure 12-14

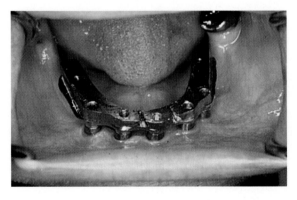

Figure 12-15

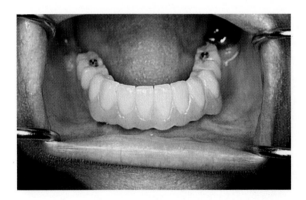

Figure 12-16

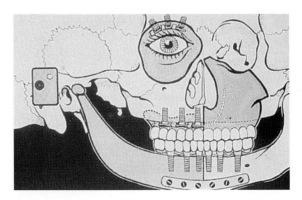

Figure 12-17

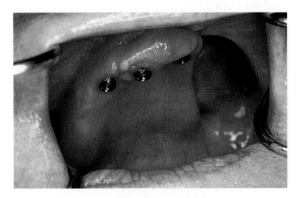

Figure 12-18

maxillary alveolus. A framework was made that incorporated three ERA coronal attachments (Figs. 12-19 and 12-20). An obturator was fabricated that engaged the attachment bar (Figs. 12-21 to 12-23). The implant-supported prosthesis gave the patient much better function. Her ability to eat a proper diet was enhanced, and her speech was greatly improved.

CLEFT PALATE REHABILITATION

Cleft palate patients have functional defects that are similar to those of the maxillectomy patient. Implant-retained prosthetics improve all oral functions, including speech, chewing,

and swallowing. The patient in Fig. 12-24 had seven implants placed to support an attachment bar that could incorporate CEKA coronal attachments (Figs. 12-25 and 12-26). The obturator encompassed the male portion of the attachment system (Figs. 12-27 and 12-28). The finished prosthesis is seen in Fig. 12-29.

CRANIOFACIAL PROSTHETICS

Bone outside the oral cavity has capabilities for osseointegration similar to those of intraoral bone. Patients with acquired or congenital craniofacial defects can benefit from implant placement also. Plastic surgery provides the ideal recon-

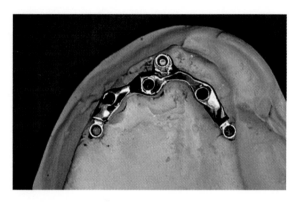

Figure 12-19

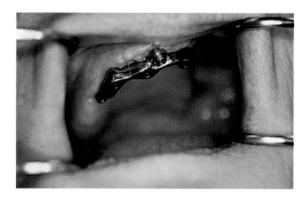

Figure 12-20

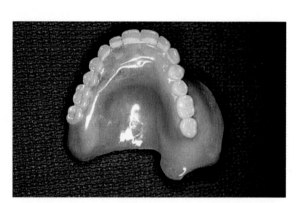

Figure 12-21

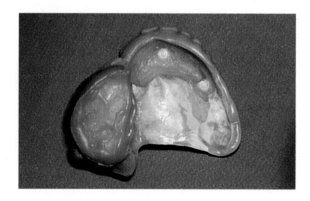

Figure 12-22

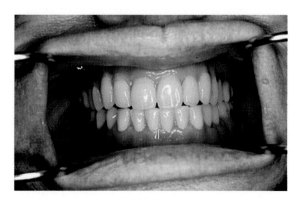

Figure 12-23

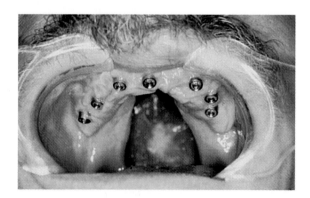

Figure 12-24

struction to correct anatomic defects; however, it has its limits as far as esthetic replacement for craniofacial defects is concerned. Fig. 12-30 shows auricular reconstruction after eight surgical procedures. Prosthetic replacements provide a more esthetic result. Scarring and pain from multiple grafting procedures are eliminated using implant-retained prosthetics.

The patient in Fig. 12-31 has hemifacial microsomia. The right ear remnant is seen in relation to implant position. Three implants were integrated, but only two were used because the third implant was in the hairline and was not essential for retention. Impressions were made, and a gold bar was fabricated using traditional components (Fig. 12-32). An

acrylic framework was used to house three gold clips. The ear was waxed on the master cast, incorporating the acrylic matrix with clips. The ear was invested, and intrinsically stained silicone was processed in the mold (Fig. 12-34). The finished auricular prosthesis is seen in Figs. 12-35 to 12-37.

Extrinsic staining was completed before prosthetic delivery. The implant-retained prosthesis has several advantages over an adhesive-retained prosthesis. Stability and retention are greatly increased with clip bar retention. Athletic pursuits are possible without dislodging the prosthesis. Patients who desire to wear an earring can do so without worrying about the ear falling off. The use of adhesives and the daily

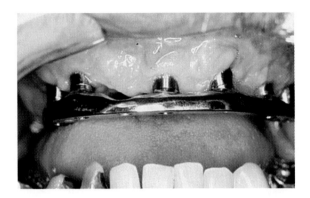

Figure 12-25

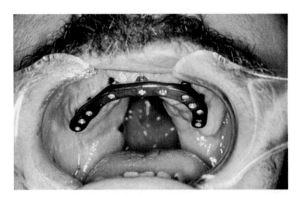

Figure 12-26

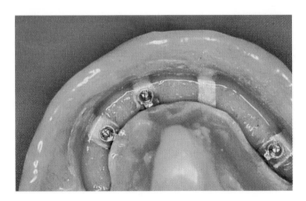

Figure 12-27

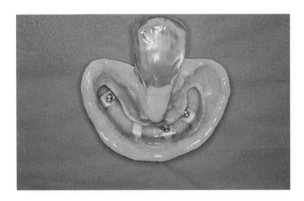

Figure 12-28

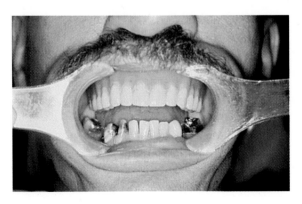

Figure 12-29

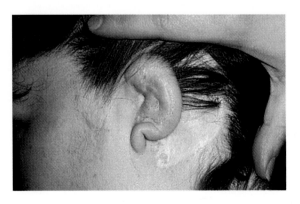

Figure 12-30

cleaning of a normal prosthesis wear down borders and the tinting may be distorted, whereas the implant-retained auricular prosthesis may last several more years without replacement. The implant-retained craniofacial prosthesis greatly enhances the patient's quality of life.

CASE REPORT: DISTRACTION OSTEOGENESIS

(This section authored by Robert Steadman)

J.H. is a 68-year-old Caucasian male patient referred by his family dentist for enucleation of a cystic-appearing lesion in the left mandible posterior region and surgical removal of adjacent second molar A.D.A. #18. Panorex radiograph showed the extent of the lesion 7 cm left posterior mandible and distal root resorption of the second molar tooth A.D.A. #18 (Fig 12-38). Surgical enucleation of the lesion and removal of A.D.A. #18 were discussed with the patient, and his informed consent was obtained. Preoperative history and a physical examination were unremarkable except for a sensitivity to certain forms of adhesive tape and borderline hypertension. The patient was not currently taking any medications.

Initial Biopsy and Pathologist Report

10/28/96: The patient was admitted to the day surgery department of the hospital, and enucleation of the 7 cm left

mandible lesion and surgical removal of A.D.A. #18 were accomplished under general anesthesia (Fig. 12-39). Clinically, the lesion was seen to be bilocular and had eroded though the lingual plate. The patient's recovery proceeded very well.

A few days later, the pathologist's report was received. The pathologist interpreted the tissue as an ameloblastoma composed of irregular nests of cells showing palisaded ameloblasts with central stellate reticulum cells. The pattern was variable from one area to another because of interdigitating nests of tumor, which frequently formed a complex pattern.

The pathology report results were discussed with the patient, including the risk of recurrence of the ameloblastoma. Surgical resection and possible alternative treatments were reviewed with the patient in detail, and his informed consent was obtained. The patient chose resection with application of a reconstruction bone plate. The patient elected not to undertake immediate bone grafting. The process of distraction osteogenesis was discussed with the patient.

Definitive Mandible Resection

1/13/97: The patient was admitted to the hospital, and resection of the left mandible ameloblastoma as accomplished (Fig. 12-40). A Synthes brand reconstruction bone plate was placed in the buccal cortex of the mandible from the proximal mandible segment across the resected area to the anterior mandible, contoured, and then removed. The first and

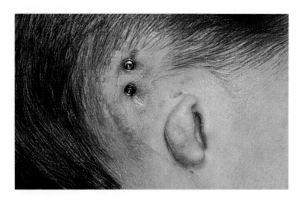

Figure 12-31

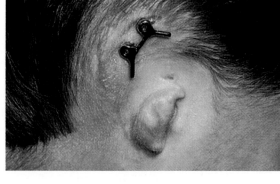

Figure 12-32

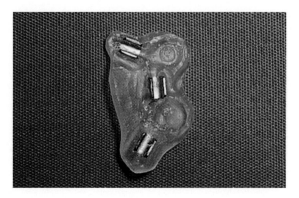

Figure 12-33

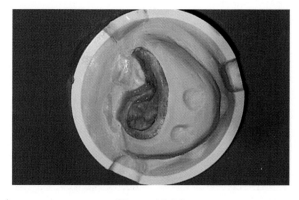

Figure 12-34

second premolars and the first molar were removed. A soft tissue excision was designed to encompass the lingual region of eroded tissue. The bony osteotomy distal was completed from the coronoid notch area inferiorly to the mandibular angle in a vertical subcondylar style osteotomy with a width of 11 mm from the posterior mandible. The anterior vertical bony osteotomy was completed distal to the second premolar region. The soft tissue incisions were completed, and the resected specimen was delivered. The previously contoured Synthes brand reconstruction bone plate was secured on the buccal cortex of the mandible from the proximal mandible segment across the resected area to the anterior

mandible (Fig. 12-41). Occlusion was verified, and the soft tissue was closed with a small Jackson-Pratt style drain in place. The patient had a satisfactory postoperative course. The postoperative pathology report revealed margins clear of tumor.

Reconstructive Phase: Transport Distraction Osteogenesis

4/97: Distraction osteogenesis was reviewed again with the patient, as was the role of the patient and spouse in activation of the appliance on a daily basis as well as appliance hygiene.

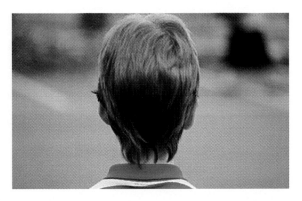

Figure 12-35

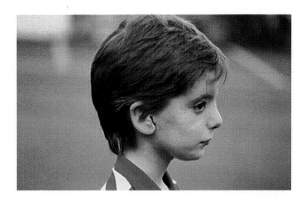

Figure 12-36

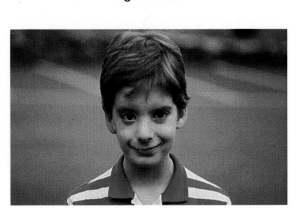

Figure 12-37

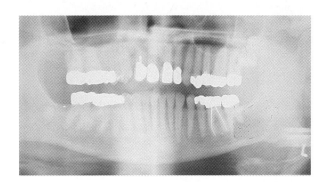

Figure 12-38

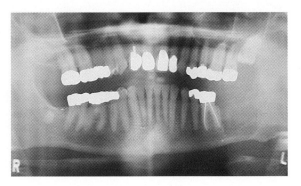

Figure 12-39

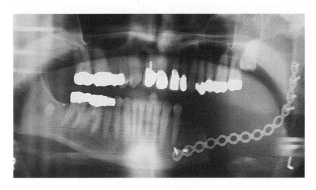

Figure 12-40

4/15/97: A KLS Martin/ACE-Normed brand multiplanar osteogenesis distractor was applied to the left mandible (Figs. 12-42 to 12-46). A transport disk of mandible bone of 16 mm thickness was created by making a vertical osteotomy through the premolar area. Two pins were applied at each fixation point engaging the anterior mandible, transport disk, and proximal condylar segment. Soft tissue was closed, and pin dressings were placed. The patient was discharged with detailed home instructions.

Appliance Activation: Distraction Osteogenesis

1. *Latency phase.* After an initial osseous and soft tissue latency healing period of 7 days, the appliance was activated. On 4/22/97, the rider stabilization screw was released and the advancement screw was turned to distract the transport disk toward the posterior resected defect 1 mm. The appliance rider stabilization screw was then secured.

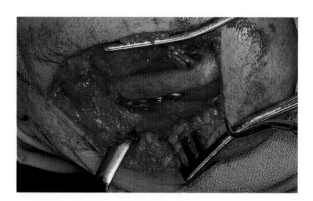

Figure 12-41

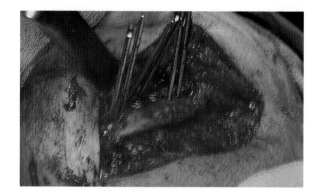

Figure 12-42

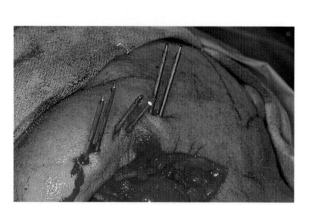

Figure 12-43

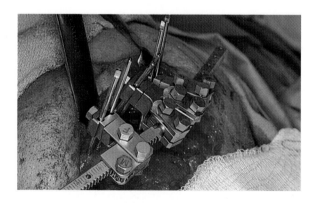

Figure 12-44

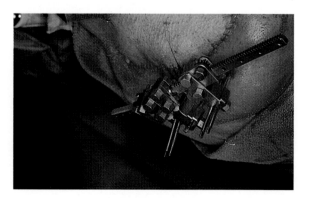

Figure 12-45

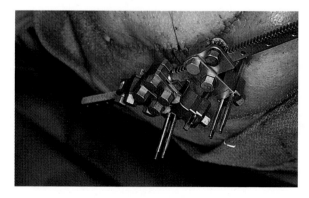

Figure 12-46

2. *Rate.* The initial activation cycle with a rate of 1.0 mm/day was completed in the office as a demonstration for the patient and his wife, and the patient's screwdriver was delivered.

3. *Rhythm.* To simplify treatment and increase compliance, a rhythm of once a day was chosen. An alternate of 0.5 mm twice-a-day rate and rhythm could have been selected. The patient was seen in the office weekly, distraction measurements were recorded, and periodic panorex radiographs were evaluated. The Synthes brand reconstruction plate served as a buccal guide for movement of the transport disk portion of the apparatus. Distraction was completed by 6/16/97, with a net gain of 55 mm osseous and soft tissue envelope (Figs 12-47 to 12-54).

4. *Fixation.* Appliance fixation was maintained until the docking procedure had been completed and a definite cortex could be visualized in the distracted bone.

Docking Procedure: Implant Stage I

9/25/97: The patient was readmitted to the hospital. The proximal posterior portion of the distracted mandible bone was exposed via a skin incision, the fibrocartilage cap was removed, the inferior ramus was exposed, and the two por-

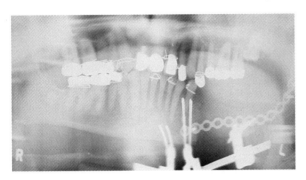

Figure 12-47

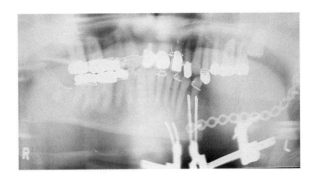

Figure 12-48

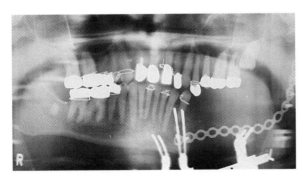

Figure 12-49

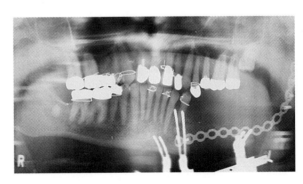

Figure 12-50

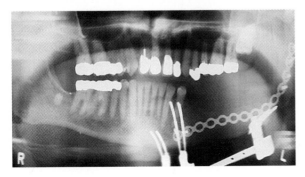

Figure 12-51

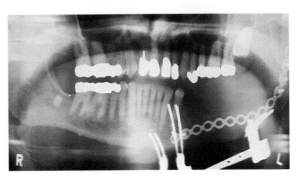

Figure 12-52

tions of the mandible were united. Small portions of iliac bone were placed to fill in small gaps and fill out contour. This completed the docking maneuver. A conservative oral incision permitted placement of three Branemark titanium dental implants anteriorly in the newly formed osteodistracted bone on the left mandible.

1. *Anterior.* 4 × 18 mm (NP) implant placed in premolar region.
2. *Middle.* 5 × 13 mm (WP) implant center point placed 7 mm posterior to (1) center.
3. *Posterior.* 5 × 13 mm (WP) implant center point placed 10 mm posterior to (2) center. Tissue was closed with 4-0 monocryl suture.

These procedures were completed under general anesthesia.

Implant Stage II and Vestibular Extension

7/20/98: The patient was admitted to the hospital, the three Branemark implants were uncovered, and 5.5 healing abutments were placed. A vestibular extension was accomplished by exposing periosteum 1 cm to buccal and lingual of implant area and placement of a 2 × 4 cm Alloderm brand acellular dermis graft. Four-millimeter fenestrations were placed in the Alloderm graft material over the implant sites.

The graft was stabilized by the projecting healing abutments and peripheral sutures. A Coe Pack brand periodontal dressing was placed (Fig 12-55). The packing was removed at 7 days (Fig 12-56). The Alloderm graft demonstrated satisfactory initial healing and placement. Permanent abutments were placed after removal of the periodontal packing:

1. Anterior 3 mm standard (NP) abutment.
2. Mid-position 2 mm (WP) abutment.
3. Posterior (WP) abutment.

Soft tissue contours were adjusted with the CO_2 laser, and the patient was prepared for prosthetic reconstruction.

Bibliography of Case Report

Abbott LC: The operative lengthening of the tibia and fibula, *J Bone Joint Surg Am* 9:125, 1927.

Annino DJ, Goguen LA, Karmody CS: Distraction osteogenesis for reconstruction of mandibular symphyseal defects, *Arch Otolaryngol Head Neck Surg* 120:911, 1994.

Block MS, Brister GD: Use of distraction osteogenesis for maxillary advancement: preliminary results, *J Oral Maxillofac Surg* 52:286, 1994.

Block MS et al: Changes in the alveolar nerve following mandibular lengthening in the dog using distraction osteogenesis, *J Oral Maxillofac Surg* 51:652, 1993.

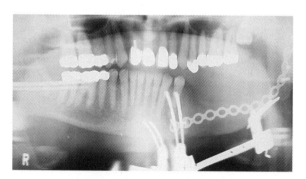

Figure 12-53

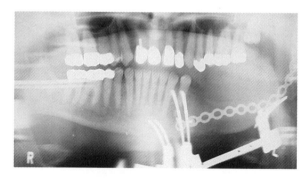

Figure 12-54

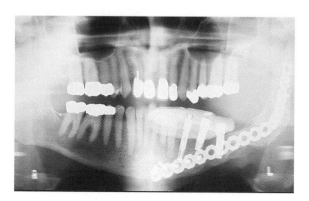

Figure 12-55

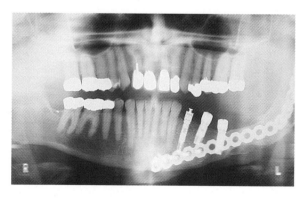

Figure 12-56

Chin M, Toth BA: Distraction osteogenesis in maxillofacial surgery using internal devices: review of five cases, *J Oral Maxillofac Surg* 54:45, 1996.

Codivilla A: On the means of lengthening in the lower limbs, the muscles and tissues which are shortened through deformity, *Am J Orthop* 2:353, 1905.

Costanio PD et al: Experimental mandibular regrowth by distraction osteogenesis, *Arch Otolaryngol Head Neck Surg* 119:511, 1993.

De Bastiani G et al: Limb lengthening by callus distraction (callotasis), *J Pediatr Orthop* 7:129, 1987.

Guerro C: Rapid mandibular expansion, *Rev Venez Ortod* 1:48, 1990.

Guerro C, Bruzual L: Application spectrum of rapid mandibular expansion, *Rev Venez Ortod* 10:170, 1993.

Guerro C, Contasti G: Transverse mandibular deficiency. In Bell WH, editor: *Modern practice in orthognathic and reconstructive surgery*, ed 3, Philadelphia, 1992, W.B. Saunders.

Ilizarov GA: A method of uniting bones in fractures and an apparatus to implement this method, *USSR Authorship Certificate* 98471, filed 1952.

Ilizarov GA: Basic principles of transosseous compression and distraction osteosynthesis, *Ortop Travmatol Protez* 32(11):7, 1971.

Ilizarov GA: The principles of the Ilizarov method, *Bull Hosp Jt Dis* 48:1, 1988.

Ilizarov GA: The tension-stress effect on the genesis of growth of tissues: Part I. The influence of stability of fixation and soft tissue preservation, *Clin Orthop* 238:249, 1989.

Ilizarov GA. The tension-stress effect on the genesis of growth of tissues: Part II. The influence of the rate and frequency of distraction, *Clin Orthop* 239:263, 1989.

Ilizarov GA, Bakhlykov YN, Petrovskaya RV: On the optimum bone formation conditions in diaphyseal thickening of the tibia (experimental study). In *Abstracts of First International Symposium on Experimental and Clinical Aspects of Transosseous Osteosynthesis*, Kurgan, USSR, September 20-22, 1983.

Ilizarov GA, Chikorina NK: Electron microscope investigation of the anterior tibial muscle in experimental tibial lengthening. In *Abstracts of First International Symposium on Experimental and Clinical Aspects of Transosseous Osteosynthesis*, Kurgan, USSR, September 20-22, 1983.

Ilizarov GA, Ledioev VI: The course of compact bone reparative regeneration in distraction osteosynthesis under different conditions of bone fragment fixation and experimental study, *Exp Khir Anest* 14:3, 1969.

Ilizarov GA, Palienko LA, Schreiner AA: The bone marrow hemopoietic function and its relationship with the activity of osteogenesis upon reparative regeneration under the conditions of crus elongation in dogs, *Ontogonez* 15:146, 1984.

Ilizarov GA et al: Blood vessels under various regimens of extremity distraction, *Anat Gistol Embryol* 86:49, 1984.

Ilizarov GA et al: On the problem of improving osteogenesis conditions in limb lengthening. In *Abstracts at First International Symposium on Experimental and Clinical Aspects of Transosseous Osteosynthesis*, Kurgan, USSR, September 20-22, 1983.

McCarthy JG et al: Lengthening the human mandible by gradual distraction, *Plast Reconstr Surg* 89:1, 1992.

McCormick SU: Osteodistraction, *Selected Readings in Oral and Maxillofacial Surgery* 4:7, 1996.

McCormick SU: Personal communication. Aisling International Boston Conference IX (Osteodistraction), Boston, Mass, Dec 11, 1996.

Michieli S, Miotti B: Lengthening of mandibular body by gradual surgical-orthodontic distraction, *J Oral Surg* 35:157, 1977.

Moore M et al: Mandibular lengthening by distraction for airway obstruction in Treacher-Collins syndrome, *J Craniofac Surg* 5:22, 1994.

Razdolsky Y et al: *Skeletal distraction of mandibular lengthening with a completely intraoral tooth borne distractor.* Submitted for publication, Moyer Craniofac Series Bk, Ann Arbor, Mich, 1998, University of Michigan.

CHAPTER 13

Procera Abutment: Computer-Generated Custom Prosthetics

Brien R. Lang
David L. Reimers

The evolution in prosthetic treatment protocols and the many designs of transmucosal components that have been introduced to the profession have been in response to resultant implant placements, functional requirements, and the esthetics demands of the patient. The number and variety of abutments available have been the direct result of the need to better orient the implant to the occlusal plane to facilitate prosthetic therapy. Implant positioning is often dictated by the anatomic features of the jaw bone and the quality and quantity of bone present. Although the surgeon has attempted to create parallelism in the placement of implants to facilitate prosthetic management, the results may not be suitable for reconstructions. Major modifications may be necessary to correct alignment through the use of transmucosal componentary, connecting the implant to the dental reconstructions.

Recently, custom abutments in titanium have entered the marketplace where an abutment can be designed by a computer and forwarded to a manufacturing facility by modem where the abutment is machined to the exact specification developed in the designing process. This new method, called the *Procera abutment* (Nobel Biocare AB, Göteborg, Sweden), provides the clinician with the opportunity to obtain an "abutment solution for every situation." The abutment is designed in one of the Nobel Biocare Network Laboratories and fabricated in a manufacturing facility remote from the laboratory. When completed, the Procera abutment is returned to the Network laboratory for finalization of the implant restoration by the dental technician.

DESIGNING THE PROCERA ABUTMENT

The Procera Cadd 3D program is part of the Procera Cadd 2D software used in the CAD/CAM process of designing and manufacturing the Procera AllCeram crown. The first screen in Procera Cadd 3D that appears on the computer provides the following command controls: (1) *Main Image*, (2) *Camera Views*, (3) *Adjust Camera*, and (4) *Main Menu* (Fig. 13-1).

The object in the window in the center of the screen in the *Main Image* is the platform, which represents either a maxillary or a mandibular cast. The abutments will be designed on this platform using several of the command buttons and "tools" specific to the program. The positioning and/or orientation of the platform and/or an object on the platform are controlled using the *Camera Views* buttons located to the left of the center screen and the *Adjust Camera* window located to the right of the center screen. The *Camera Views* and the *Adjust Camera* controls remain active throughout the various activities of the abutment program.

The *Camera Views* buttons project the various camera angles that can be activated in viewing the platform and objects in the *Main Image*. The *Adjust Camera* screen orients the position of the camera to the object on the platform in the center screen. The operator is able to rotate the camera, move the camera, and zoom in and out. The object on the platform can be viewed in low, medium, or high resolution by pressing the *Redraw* button located in the *Adjust Camera* window.

The *Main Menu* located in the bottom portion of this first screen lists the different functions within the program (Fig. 13-2). All of the functions are used during some aspect of the design process. The *Object Module System* is used in selecting the abutment for a given location (Figs. 13-3 and 13-4). The *Move Object* menu is used to align the implant in the dental arch (Fig. 13-5). The alignment is achieved through visualization of the spatial relationship of a special guide T-bar attached to the abutment analog of the master cast and then creating this same relationship in the virtual module on the *Move Object* screens (Fig. 13-6). The implant and abutment default objects that appear on the *Move Object* screens can be moved horizontally and vertically using those adjustment buttons. The default position of the abutment can be rotated using the *Rotate T-Bar* button until the position of the virtual T-bar on the screen is as close as possible to the position of the physical T-bar on the master cast.

When a match of the virtual alignment and the actual alignment on the master cast has been completed, the *Abutment Design* menu is selected from the *Main Menu* (Fig. 13-7). These screens provide adjustment of the width and height of the abutment collar in both the mesial/distal and facial/lingual directions. The abutment collar can be tilted, and the finish line can be raised or lowered to create the appropriate emergence profile. The body of the abutment can also be bodily moved horizontally right or left, increased or decreased in width, tilted, and adjusted in height. Guide scales are available to assist the operator in designing the

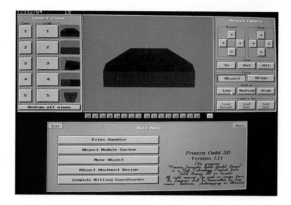

Figure 13-1

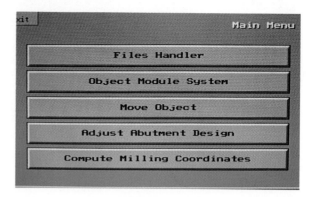

Figure 13-2

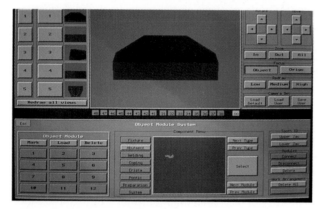

Figure 13-3

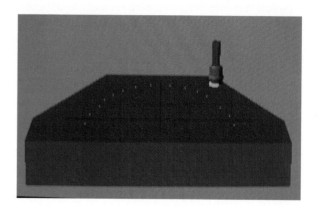

Figure 13-4

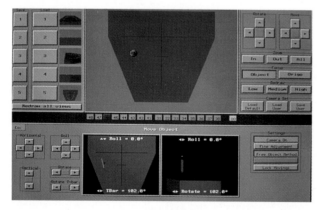

Figure 13-5

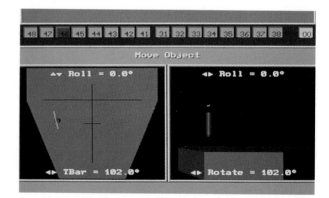

Figure 13-6

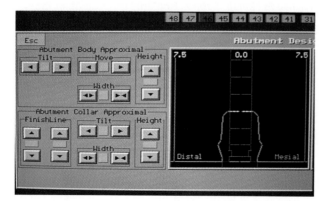

Figure 13-7

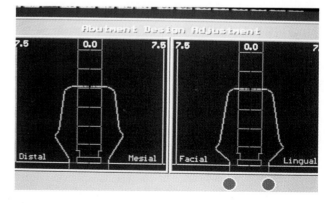

Figure 13-8

abutment collar, body, and overall height. If the angle formed below the finish line is too steep, a red dot appears on the screen indicating that an adjustment is needed to correct the design (Fig. 13-8).

Finally, the Procera abutment design is saved to a file using the *Files Handler* menu, which also prepares the data for transfer by modem to the manufacturing facility. Within a few days the finished Procera abutment is returned to the laboratory, and the finalization of the restoration is completed.

ADVANTAGES OF THE PROCERA ABUTMENT

The Procera abutment created by the Cadd program mates precisely with the implant-bearing surface. The abutment allows development of the ideal emergence profile and a machined external surface. The custom abutment accommodates cementable prosthetics and can be directly linked to Procera AllCeram restorations. Through the Cadd program the positioning of the finish line at the exact location for esthetics and the proper restoration contours is possible.

Problems, Complications, and Solutions

Implant prosthodontics can be straightforward when fixture position and angulation are ideal. If prosthetic components are used properly and framework design and fit are perfect, complications can be minimized. Component and framework breakage, inadequate tissue support, poor implant position and angulation, and implant loss complicate prosthetic treatment and may compromise the prosthetic result. This chapter discusses complications with implant rehabilitation and possible causes and solutions for the complications.

COMPONENT AND FRAMEWORK DESIGN

The reasons for gold and abutment screw loosening and fracture are as follows:

1. Screw design
2. Inadequate torque application
3. Cantilever extension
4. Inaccurate framework abutment interface
5. Occlusal discrepancy and jaw relationship
6. Implant position and arch form

Screw Design

Conical screws were originally used for framework retention (Fig. 14-1). These screws have a tendency to loosen. Torque applied through handheld screwdrivers was used for tightening. Hand strength varies between dentists, and incomplete tightening or binding on the conical screw head caused occasional loosening of the screws and therefore loosening of the prosthesis. An increase in prosthesis movement applied torque to implant components and contributed to component loosening and breakage. The gold screw and gold cylinder have been redesigned, and a flat-head screw is now used. The force of torquing the screw is now incorporated into the threads, and the inadvertent loosening of properly torqued flat-head screws is rare (Fig. 14-2). These screws are weaker than conical screws, and excessive hand torquing can induce stress fractures or actually fracture the screws.

Inadequate Torque Application

A mechanical torque driver has been developed to ensure proper tightening (Figs. 14-3 and 14-4). Recommended torque for prosthetic gold screws is 10 Ncm, and 20 Ncm is recommended for the abutment screw. A manual torque converter is available to adjust between 10 Ncm and 20 Ncm. Another torque driver has been developed that is electric and is adjustable to 32 Ncm for the CeraOne system, 20 Ncm for abutment screws, and 10 Ncm for gold screws (Figs. 14-5 and 14-6). It is recommended that all screws be tightened with a torque driver. The wide-platform components and larger-diameter implants discussed in Chapter 9 were designed to allow higher torque application. The torque drivers are expensive, and many practitioners have been lax in the use of this equipment. *Proper torque is mandatory in all implant prosthetics.* Patients are advised at the prosthetic delivery appointment and during hygiene recall appointments to monitor for prosthesis loosening. Abut-ments with a visual framework abutment interface are checked for looseness by observing the interface while grasping the incisors and attempting to move the prosthesis. If movement is present, saliva can be seen percolating at the interface. If movement is detectable clinically, the gold screws are accessed and checked for tightness. The prosthesis is removed, and all components are examined. If any of the gold screws are loose, all should be replaced. Undetectable stress fractures may be present in previously used screws if prosthesis movement is present. Broken gold or abutment screws may be evident when the prosthesis is removed (Figs. 14-7 to 14-9). The remaining shaft is removed from the abutment screw using hemostats if adequate length exists for engagement. An explorer tip that is used in a counterclockwise direction on the screw shaft also may work. A slowly rotating #0.5 bur or a #1 round bur in a slow-speed handpiece is used for shafts that are broken close to the abutment screw head. When a loose prosthesis is removed, abutment screws may be fractured. The junction of the abutment screw head and shaft is where fracture usually occurs. The same methods for gold screw removal are used for abutment screw shaft removal. Individual abutment screws are available and are used with the original abutment, unless it has been damaged; this will ensure that the old prosthesis will fit the same as it did before the screw fractured. If total abutment replacement is necessary, the same length abutment is used, the original prosthesis is positioned, and the interfaces are checked (as described previously). Rarely, the gold screw slot may be distorted by repeated loosening and tightening, preventing removal of the screw. The screw head can be reslotted, if accessible, or the head of the screw can be severed from the shank with a dental bur (Figs. 14-10 to 14-12).

Arch Form

Bracing support created by cross-arch splinting when implants are used to restore the edentulous mandible resists the lateral forces transmitted to the joints between implant and abutment and abutment prosthesis. When an arch form is maintained, a tripod effect lessens bending moments transmitted to the screw joints. Fig. 14-7 shows a straight-line arrangement of implant abutments minimizing the beneficial tripod effects. The destructive forces cause loosening of the prosthetic and abutment screws as well as fracture of the screws (see Figs. 14-7 to 14-9). Prosthetic movement may cause the hexagonal heads of the abutment screws to wear, making use of the hexagonal wrench impossible. Occasionally an impression guide pin can be screwed into the hole in the abutment screw designed for the prosthetic screw and torqued to 20 NdC. Reversing the torque driver may allow backing out of the abutment screw (Figs. 14-13 and 14-14).

The use of a high-speed handpiece with an inverted cone or small round bur may allow slotting and removal of the

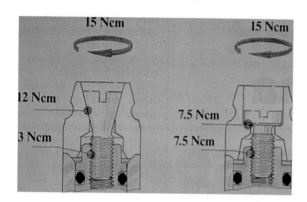

Figure 14-1

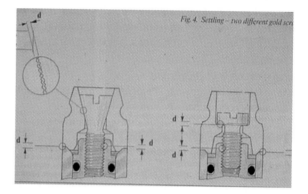

Figure 14-2

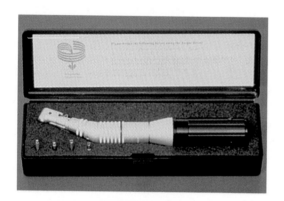

Figure 14-3

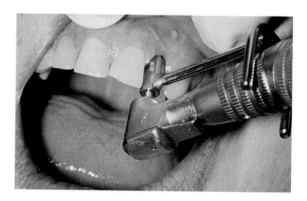

Figure 14-4

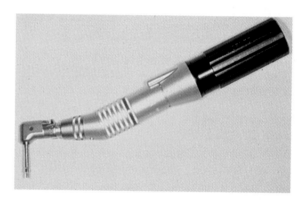

Figure 14-5

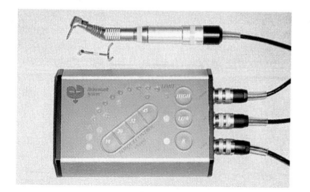

Figure 14-6

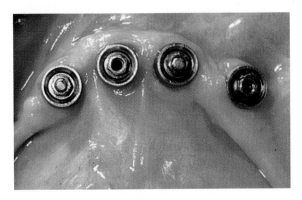

Figure 14-7

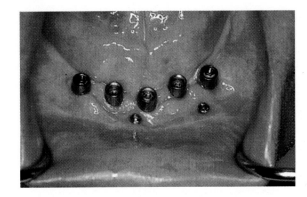

Figure 14-8

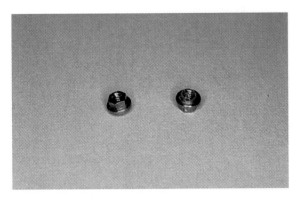

Figure 14-9

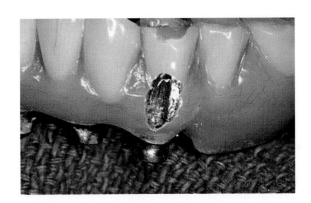

Figure 14-10

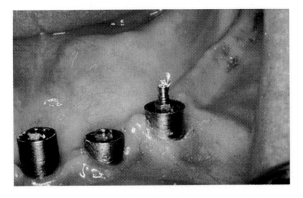

Figure 14-11

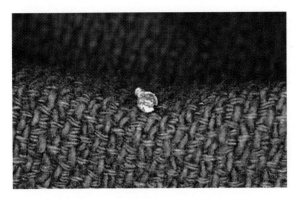

Figure 14-12

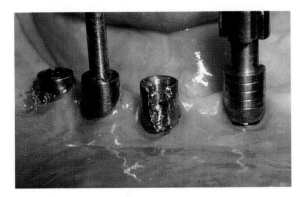

Figure 14-13

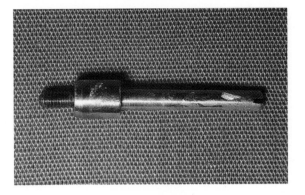

Figure 14-14

abutment screw. Broken heads of abutment screws may allow burnishing of the metal and make screw removal impossible. Splitting the abutment with the appropriate burs will allow abutment removal (see Fig. 14-13). Care must be taken not to damage the implant itself.

Fig. 14-13 shows a combination of loose and broken components, including an abutment that needed to be split for removal. Six hours were needed to remove and replace components, but the existing prosthesis fit well with new components (Figs. 14-15 and 14-16).

Similar problems were much more common in posterior implant prosthetics because of lack of arch form and fewer implants to provide the tripod effect. The lack of arch form was complicated by a cantilever distance of 20 mm (Fig. 14-17) that used to be recommended for fixed prosthetics on five mandibular implants.

Implant Loss

Implant loss rarely occurs after prosthetic completion. If implant loss occurs in fixed prosthetics in an edentulous arch, conversion to an overdenture may be completed and an additional implant placed for later conversion back to fixed prosthetics.

Occasionally very poor treatment planning and treatment may result in disasters as seen in Figs. 14-18 to 14-20. A panoramic radiograph shows 7 mm implants placed in an extremely resorbed mandible. A 3:1 abutment prosthesis to implant thread ratio is seen in Fig. 14-19. Four extremely retentive metal clips were used to retain the mandibular overdenture. Retention made this prosthesis similar to a fixed restoration. Opposing natural dentition only complicated the situation. This is a prime example of very poor treatment planning and execution and would have made a fine malpractice case.

Occasionally, implant movement will not be detected by the surgeon at the abutment surgery. When temporary healing abutments are removed by the restorative dentist, the implant may unscrew with the healing abutment, as seen in Fig. 14-21.

Implant Fracture

The traditional implant, abutment, and prosthesis unit involves two screws. The abutment screw holds the abutment to the implant, and the prosthetic screws hold the prosthesis to the abutments. Both screws are designed with breakaway points. The goal of this system is to preserve and protect the implant while allowing replaceable components to break before the implants. The UCLA-type abutment was designed to compensate for lack of intermaxillary space and to improve esthetics in certain situations. Although absolutely necessary in certain clinical situations, the UCLA-type abutment bypasses the failsafe of the two-screw system. Since the junc-

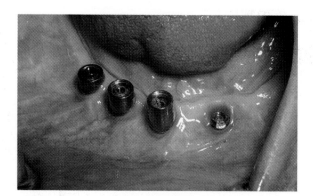

Figure 14-15

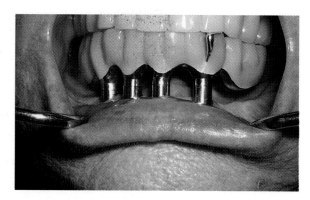

Figure 14-16

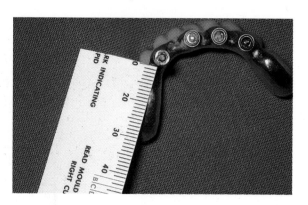

Figure 14-17

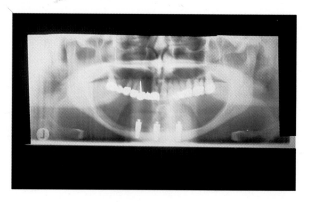

Figure 14-18

tion between the prosthesis and implant is below tissue, the fit of the framework can only be checked radiographically, which may lead to poor-fitting frameworks. Overload may cause implant fracture. To date, the practice of the authors has re-stored thousands of implants with four implant fractures. All four involved the UCLA-type abutment. The authors believe that the two-screw system with failsafes should be used if at all possible. Larger-diameter implants with wide platforms and larger screws that can be torqued to higher specifications should minimize complications (see Chapter 9). An overdenture bar was directly attached to the implants in Fig. 14-22. Swelling is seen where implant fractures occurred. The fractured components are seen in Fig. 14-23.

Cantilever Extension

The cantilevered distance beyond the distal implant determines the lever arm length and the amount of force that is transmitted to the implants, framework, and components. A length of 20 mm of cantilever was originally recommended for the fixed mandibular prosthesis on four or more implants. Several factors may modify cantilever length, including implant length, arch form, spacing, bone quality, occlusal considerations, and parafunctional habits. More research is needed to determine cantilever length for each situation. It is recommended that the cantilever length on five or more implants in the mandible be limited to 15 mm or less and 10

mm or less in the maxilla when five or more implants are used. The modifying factors listed previously may shorten the recommended cantilever length.

Overextension of the cantilever may lead to gold screw fracture, abutment screw fracture, loosening of the prosthesis, and possibly implant loss. If an existing prosthesis has an intimately fitting framework (no occlusal discrepancies and no parafunctional habits exist) but component fracture occurs repeatedly, the cantilever length should be shortened.

Inaccurate Framework Abutment Interface

The prosthetic components are designed to specific tolerances to allow a precise junction between abutments and prosthetic frameworks. An ideal framework abutment connection is one that has circumferential contact and is without an opening at the interface. Inaccuracy in framework abutment interface will cause a constant tension on components when the gold screws are tightened to recommended torque. This constant stress may cause component loosening or breakage. Implants under tension may be sensitive for the patient, and ill-fitting frameworks may eventually cause loss of osseointegration. Therefore the framework abutment connection must be passive for long-term success. When evaluating the fit, screws should be tightened one at a time while observing the lift of the frame and the open interfaces. Torquing all the gold screws before evaluating the interface

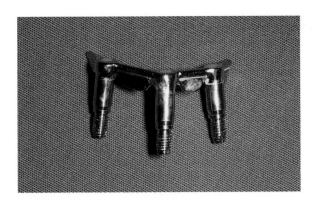

Figure 14-19

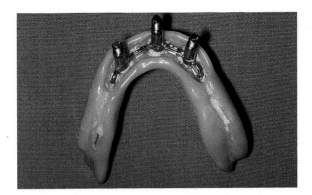

Figure 14-20

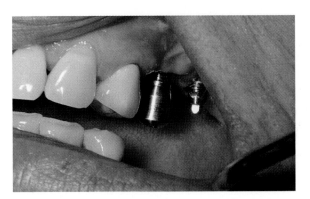

Figure 14-21

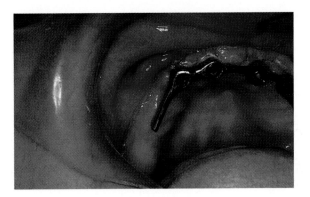

Figure 14-22

may bend the framework, giving the appearance of accuracy. Figs. 14-24 and 14-25 show reasonable visual interfacing; however, when the distal screws are loosened, the gap between the framework and the abutment opens significantly (Figs. 14-26 and 14-27). If these frames are seated, a constant stress is placed on the implants and the components, potentially causing complications. Therefore all framework fittings should be visualized before tightening all screws. Individual screws should be tightened, and the framework fit should be observed on other abutments. Any discrepancy in fit demands framework sectioning, solder indexing, soldering, and then a clinical reevaluation of the fit.

Occlusal Factors

Optimally, occlusal force should be shared equally by all implants. Although an equal distribution is rarely achieved, force distribution can be improved with careful occlusal adjustment during laboratory remounts, as well as intraorally during the delivery appointment. Shimstock is used to verify all occlusal contacts. In a Class II jaw relationship or with the implant angled or placed lingual to the ridge crest, an anterior cantilever may be present along the distal cantilever (Fig. 14-28); this will transmit additional force to the components, and an increase in component breakage may be seen.

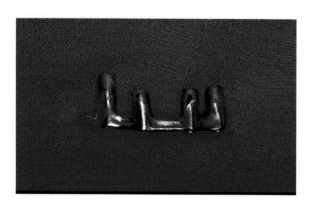

Figure 14-23

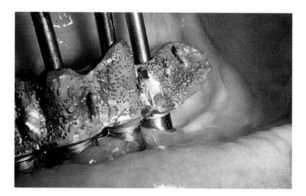

Figure 14-24

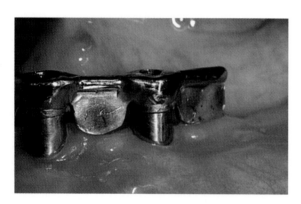

Figure 14-25

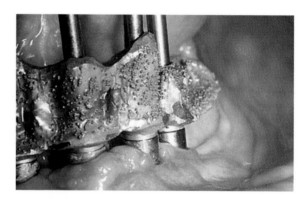

Figure 14-26

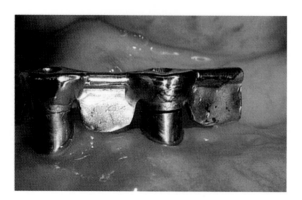

Figure 14-27

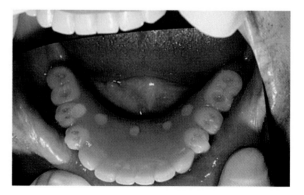

Figure 14-28

Framework Fracture

A properly designed framework should not fracture. A cross-sectional dimension of at least 4 mm × 6 mm is needed. A J-shaped beam, with the occlusal gingival height having the greater dimension, will provide strength and resist fracture. The alloy should have a tensile strength of at least 60,000 Ncm. Common areas of framework fracture are through the solder joints and just distal to the distal-most implant (Figs. 14-29 to 14-37). Because of the cantilever, this region is subjected to a higher force, and an adequate cross-sectional dimension is needed to resist fracture. Improperly soldered joints also are subject to fracture (see Figs. 14-29 to 14-33).

Fractured solder joints may be reindexed intraorally and then soldered. The heat of soldering will destroy any acrylic veneering material; this is replaced after the framework fit has been verified after soldering. A framework fracture caused by a minimal cross-sectional dimension in the metal may require a frame remake.

TISSUE SUPPORT

Alveolar resorption or trauma may leave an inadequate amount of alveolar bone, thereby leaving patients with an inadequate tissue contour to support an implant-retained prosthesis. Complete dentures compensate for bone loss,

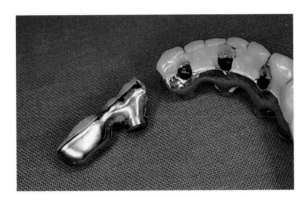

Figure 14-29

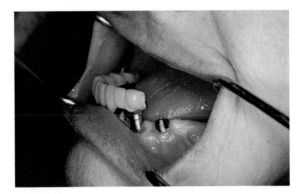

Figure 14-30

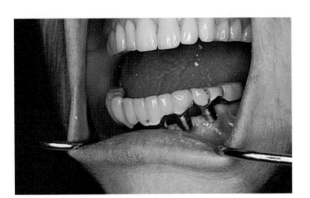

Figure 14-31

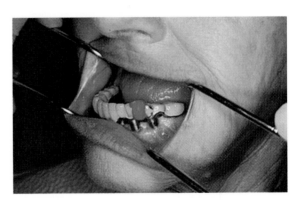

Figure 14-32

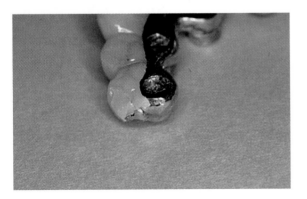

Figure 14-33

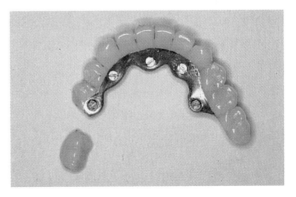

Figure 14-34

with the denture flange providing tissue support. Patients wearing conventional prosthetics may be accustomed to ideal or excess tissue support provided by the flange, especially in the mentolabial fold and nasolabial fold. An implant-supported fixed prosthesis may not provide tissue support or esthetically acceptable contours in these areas. The alternatives for use in the mandible are an implant-retained overdenture or a gingival insert (Figs. 14-38 to 14-41). In the maxilla, bone grafting may provide ideal contours. An over-denture or gingival insert may esthetically compensate for bone loss. The overdenture technique is described in Chapter 10.

GINGIVAL INSERT

The insert is created by making an impression of the completed fixed prosthesis. A vinyl polysiloxane putty is mixed and placed in the labial vestibule. It should cover the labial side of the prosthesis to the floor of the vestubule. The mate-

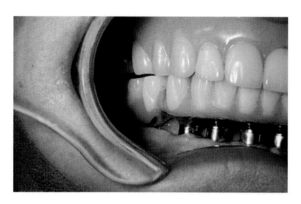

Figure 14-35

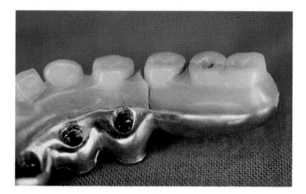

Figure 14-36

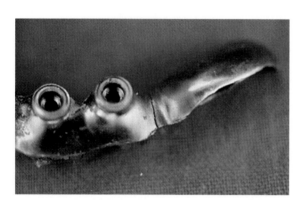

Figure 14-37

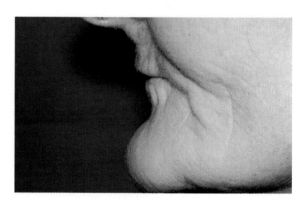

Figure 14-38

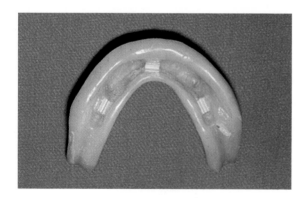

Figure 14-39

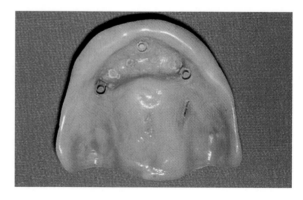

Figure 14-40

rial should be pressed between the abutments and should cover the distal buccal extent of the prosthesis. After the material has set, the putty matrix is removed. Injection viscosity vinyl polysiloxane impression material is placed in a thin layer on the lingual surface of the putty, and the matrix is positioned back in the mouth. The impression is removed after it has set and is poured in diestone (Fig. 14-42 and 14-43). A wax pattern is made on the master cast (Fig. 14-44). The cast is invested, boiled out, and may be packed with a soft reline material or methylmethacrylate resin (Figs. 14-45 to 14-48). The cast will be destroyed with the methylmethacrylate resin, and a duplicate cast that is made before investing is used for adjustments and for a proper path of insertion.

IMPLANT POSITION AND ANGULATION

Poor planning, lack of adequate bone, or poor surgical technique may leave implants and abutments in a less-than-ideal

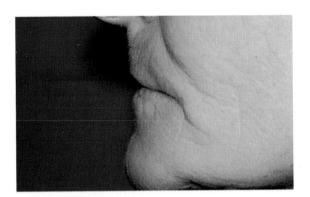

Figure 14-41

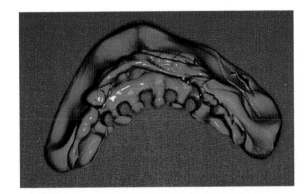

Figure 14-42

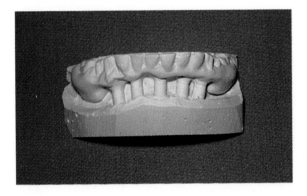

Figure 14-43

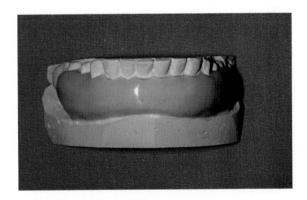

Figure 14-44

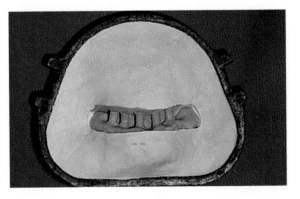

Figure 14-45

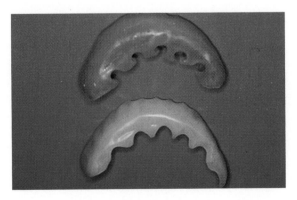

Figure 14-46

position. Esthetics, phonetics, hygiene, and prosthetic design may be compromised by poor implant position (Figs. 14-49 to 14-53). In severe cases, the implants may not be usable at all and may have to be removed or left in the bone without abutment placement. Components have been developed that compensate for poor implant angulation (Figs. 14-53 to 14-57). The angulated abutments are designed to change the abutment angulation by either 17 or 30 degrees. In turn this changes the screw access direction by 17 or 30 degrees. This change in angulation eliminates prosthetic compromise in most situations. A 17-degree angulated abutment is available also.

The angulated abutment has 12 facets and 12 positions of angulation in a 360-degree circle. It is recommended that the prosthodontist place the angulated abutment to ensure the best possible angulation. The surgeon often will not know which direction is best for restoring the patient (Fig. 14-58). Fig. 14-59 shows the angulated abutments in the ideal posi-

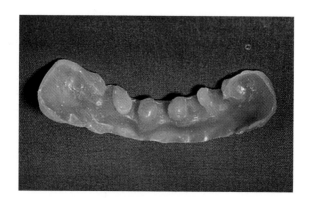

Figure 14-47

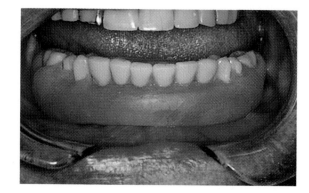

Figure 14-48

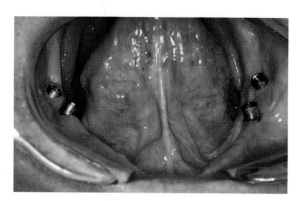

Figure 14-49

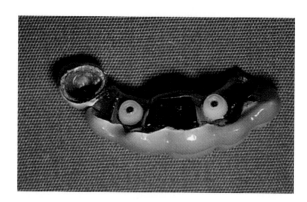

Figure 14-50

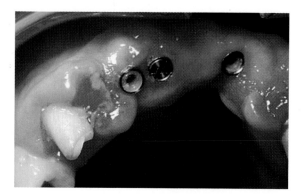

Figure 14-51

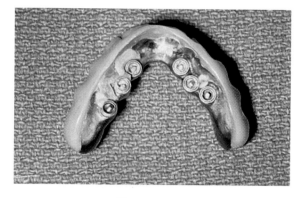

Figure 14-52

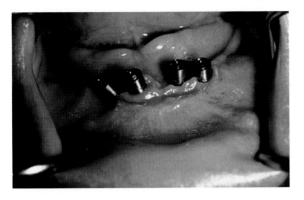

Figure 14-53

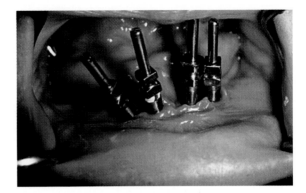

Figure 14-54

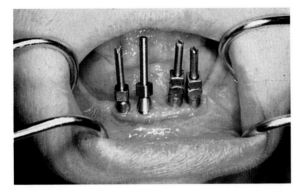

Figure 14-55

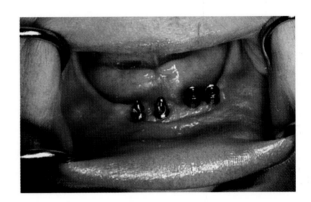

Figure 14-56

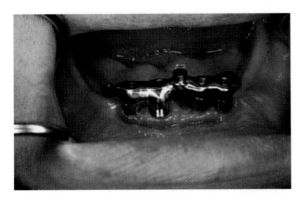

Figure 14-57

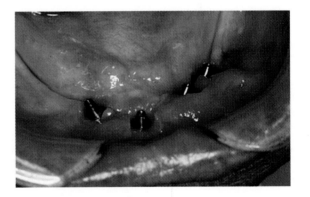

Figure 14-58

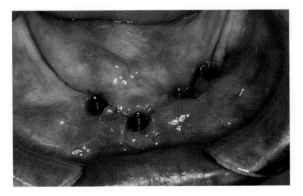

Figure 14-59

tion. A system of impression copings, gold cylinders, laboratory analogues, and healing caps have been developed for use with the angulated abutment.

Labially tipped abutments may have a screw access hole that exits through the labial veneering material or through the incisal edge; this compromises the strength and esthetics of the veneer. Excess labial angulation and position may interfere with normal denture flange position with an implant-retained overdenture (Figs. 14-60 to 14-62). Lingual or palatal angulation may encroach on the neutral zone and interfere with speech (Figs. 14-63 and 14-64).

In the maxillary anterior, the collar of the angulated abutment may compromise esthetics or oral hygiene (Figs. 14-65 to 14-69). This problem can be minimized if adequate bone exists for countersinking the implant enough to have the abutment collar below tissue. Most angulation and position

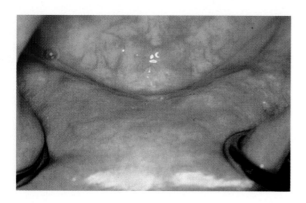

Figure 14-60

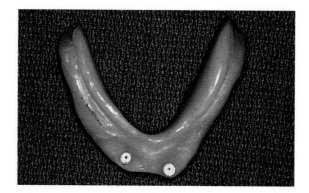

Figure 14-61

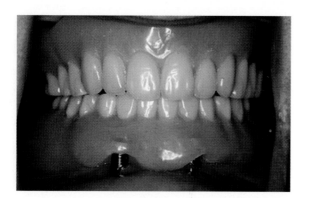

Figure 14-62

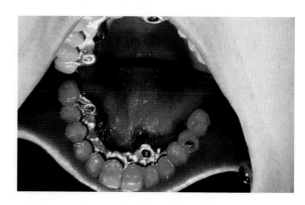

Figure 14-63

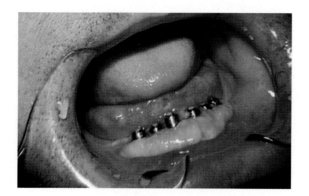

Figure 14-64

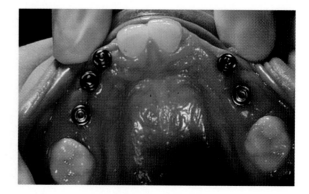

Figure 14-65

problems can be eliminated by careful treatment planning and communication between the restorative dentist, the oral surgeon, and the dental technician, as well as by the use of a surgical stent.

Most complications are a result of poor existing anatomy before implant placement, poor treatment planning or execution, or mechanical problems caused by components that are too small or torque requirements that limit the joint tightness between the implant, abutment, and prosthetic framework. Chapter 9 discusses the use and indications for larger components, which allow for higher torque application and increased resistance to loosening or breakage. In Chapter 5 and elsewhere, modifying the existing anatomy with bone grafting, and even with orthognathic surgery, is discussed.

Many new components are available on the market with claims that they simplify technique and lower costs for dentists. Cementable prosthetics are being used at an alarming rate. The problems associated with new components and techniques with little to no clinical trial research promises to make the complications multiply. Proven techniques well documented for years exist to handle complications and min-imize them, but economically driven sales and untested components promise to confuse restorative dentists and provide a multitude of complications in the future.

Cementable prosthetics, especially for multiple-implant restorations, will not be predictably retrievable for repair, whereas screw-retained prosthetics are always retrievable. The authors have documented and "rescued" hundreds of implant complications. Some problems are inevitable when the restorative dentist has restored over 1000 patients, but the authors' complications in private practice are now minimal and easily remedied at a reasonable expense. The patients that the authors see now are referred from other dentists, and more than 90% have cementable implant prosthetics.

Most of these patients need to have the cementable prosthetics cut off, destroyed, and, remade. Most of these patients have had their implant restorations for less than 5 years and are understandably upset for having to pay thousands of dollars again for new prosthetics. The authors advise against cementable prosthetics unless absolutely necessary, and patients should be made more aware of options and sign consent forms before the work has begun.

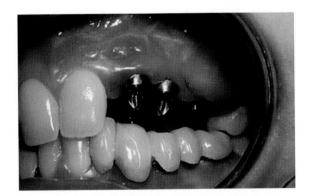

Figure 14-66

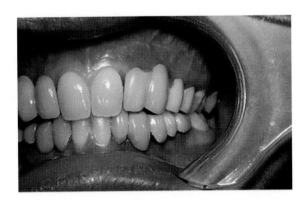

Figure 14-67

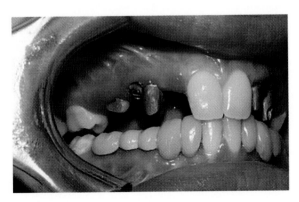

Figure 14-68

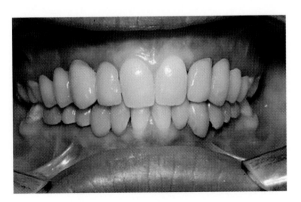

Figure 14-69

Chapter 15

Hygiene and Maintenance Guidelines

Deborah L. Steele
Gayle S. Orton

Diligent and precise surgical and prosthetic procedures are critical to the success of implant therapy, but maintenance of implants may be of equal importance in ensuring a long-term, favorable prognosis. The dental professional's responsibility in providing supportive therapy and education in maintaining dental implants is crucial. This chapter defines the clinician's responsibilities in examining and assessing the tissues surrounding the transmucosal abutment, as well as the implant and its supporting prosthesis. Suggestions for the removal of hard and soft deposits, recommendations for home care procedures, and guidelines for appropriate professional maintenance intervals are included.

EXAMINATION OF THE PERI-IMPLANT TISSUES AND PROSTHESIS

Examination and assessment of the soft tissues surrounding the dental implant abutment and prosthesis provide the clinician with valuable information that may influence treatment planning. For example, the presence of hard and soft deposits and the current status of the peri-implant tissues will influence the kind and type of individualized home care instructions that must be offered.

Clinical assessment of peri-implant soft tissues begins with a visual examination. Characteristics of the soft tissue, including tone, color, contour, size, and consistency, should be noted and compared with baseline records. The presence of inflamed or exuberant tissues should be documented and correlated with the presence of hard and soft deposits. Various maintenance record forms may be used for this purpose (Fig. 15-1). Clinicians may find it useful to record the presence or absence of keratinized tissues immediately surrounding a transmucosal abutment. As long as good oral hygiene levels are maintained, tissue health is probably not dependent on the existence of keratinized tissues. However, nonkeratinized tissue surrounding abutments may create a condition that is sensitive to the patient, influencing his or her ability to keep the abutment cylinders free of deposits.

The issue of routine probing for clinical assessment of the peri-implant tissues is currently being debated. Baseline probe readings may be recorded at the time of prosthesis delivery and before the appliance is seated. Thereafter, in the absence of pain, discomfort, or other clinical signs of disease

(inflamed or exuberant tissues, mobility, or bone loss), the value of probing may be questioned. Appropriate clinical judgment must be used in determining the need for probing. In any case, probing of the sulcus, if performed, must be atraumatic. If multiple abutments are connected by a prosthetic suprastructure, obtaining accurate probe readings may be difficult because of access problems in positioning the probe tip parallel to the long axis of the transmucosal abutment. Flexible plastic probes may reduce this problem; however, the most accurate readings are obtained when the suprastructure is removed.

Absolute probe readings and attachment levels are not as critical in terms of the success or failure of an implant as are progressive changes in either of these two parameters over time. The average depth of the peri-implant sulcus varies because of several factors. Examples include abutment height, depth of implant countersinking at stage 1 surgery, and the amount of tissue thinning during stage 2 surgery procedures. There may be instances in which the probing depth is greater than 4 mm and yet is still associated with a healthy, stable implant. Thicker fibrotic tissues, such as those located in the palatal region, provide a good example.

After the soft tissue has been assessed and documented, the presence or absence of mobility of the implants, the transmucosal abutments, and the prosthetic suprastructure should be evaluated. Many clinicians routinely remove the prosthesis yearly to definitively test for implant and abutment mobility; others remove the suprastructure only if clinical signs and symptoms warrant the procedure. Since a successful osseointegrated implant has no periodontal ligament, zero mobility is anticipated around stable implants.

The absence of a periodontal ligament precludes the ability of the implant to absorb any excess loading. Occlusal trauma of any magnitude from the prosthesis will negatively influence the surrounding supporting structures of the implant and may lead to their destruction. If any mobility is present, optimal occlusion cannot be obtained. To check for mobility of the suprastructure, two instrument handles or the thumb and index finger of one hand can be used to attempt to physically move the prosthesis (Fig. 15-2). The clinician should be alert for the presence of salivary percolation at the interface where the prosthesis meets the coronal portion of the abutment cylinder. Small bubbles of saliva usually indi-

Brånemark system®
Maintenance record

Patient's name _____

Chart # _____   Referring Dr. _____   Alternate recalls Y / N

Medical alert	Maintenance interval	Next appointment

Months 2   Minutes 30   1. _____

                             3   45   2. _____

                             4   60   3. _____

                             6   90   4. _____

Charting code (cc)*

B-Bleeding	M-Mobility
C-Calculus	N-Normal
D-Discharge/suppuration	NK-Nonkeratinized
E-Edematous, soft	P-Plaque
F-Fibrous enlargement	R-Redness
K-Keratinized	S-Sensitivity

Special considerations: _____

_____

_____

_____

_____

Date _____

DDS√: Y /N   Fee: _____

Changes

Medical history   Y / N _____

Dental history   Y / N _____

EO/IO exam   Y / N _____

Radiographs: (type)

Procedures performed

Tissue assessment   Y / N

Prosthesis removed   Y / N

Calculus removed   Y / N

Coronal polish   Y / N

Home care instructions

Recommended: _____

_____

_____

Uses: _____

_____

_____

Patient compliance: good/poor

Comments: _____

_____

_____

Signature: _____

Probing depths (of natural teeth)

	1-8	1-7	1-6	1-5	1-4	1-3	1-2	1-1	2-1	2-2	2-3	2-4	2-5	2-6	2-7	2-8
Fa																
*cc																
Li																
*cc																

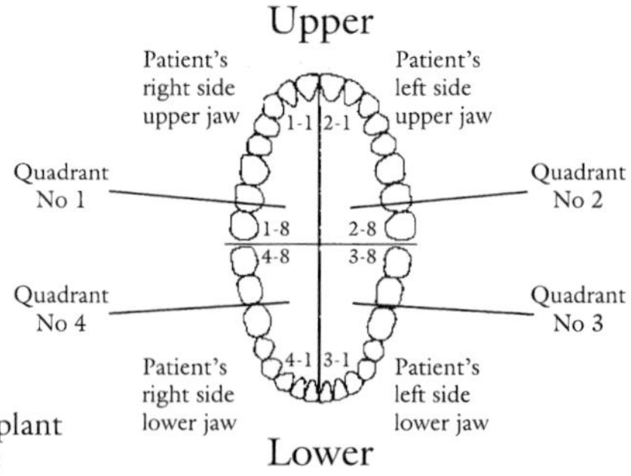

Upper

Patient's right side upper jaw

Patient's left side upper jaw

Quadrant No 1

Quadrant No 2

Quadrant No 4

Quadrant No 3

Patient's right side lower jaw

Patient's left side lower jaw

Designate implant abutment site in blue

Lower

	4-8	4-7	4-6	4-5	4-4	4-3	4-2	4-1	3-1	3-2	3-3	3-4	3-5	3-6	3-7	3-8
Li																
*cc																
Fa																
*cc																

Figure 15-1

Date _____
DDS√: Y / N   Fee: _____

Changes
Medical history Y / N _____
Dental history   Y / N _____
EO/IO exam   Y / N _____
Radiographs: (type)

Procedures performed
Tissue assessment   Y / N
Prosthesis removed Y / N
Calculus removed   Y / N
Coronal polish   Y / N

Home care instructions

Recommended: _____

_____

_____

Uses: _____

_____

Patient compliance: good/poor

Comments: _____

_____

_____

Signature: _____

Probing Depths (of natural teeth)

	1-8	1-7	1-6	1-5	1-4	1-3	1-2	1-1	2-1	2-2	2-3	2-4	2-5	2-6	2-7	2-8
Fa																
*cc																
Li																
*cc																

Upper

Patient's right side upper jaw   Patient's left side upper jaw

Quadrant No 1   1-1 2-1   Quadrant No 2

1-8   2-8
4-8   3-8

Quadrant No 4   Quadrant No 3

Patient's right side lower jaw   4-1 3-1   Patient's left side lower jaw

Designate implant abutment site in blue

Lower

	4-8	4-7	4-6	4-5	4-4	4-3	4-2	4-1	3-1	3-2	3-3	3-4	3-5	3-6	3-7	3-8
Li																
*cc																
Fa																
*cc																

Date _____
DDS√: Y /N   Fee: _____

Changes
Medical history   Y / N _____
Dental history   Y / N _____
EO/IO exam   Y / N _____
Radiographs: (type)

Procedures performed

Tissue assessment   Y / N
Prosthesis removed   Y / N
Calculus removed   Y / N
Coronal polish   Y / N

Home care instructions

Recommended: _____

_____

_____

Uses: _____

_____

Patient compliance: good/poor

Comments: _____

_____

_____

Signature: _____

Probing Depths (of natural teeth)

	1-8	1-7	1-6	1-5	1-4	1-3	1-2	1-1	2-1	2-2	2-3	2-4	2-5	2-6	2-7	2-8
Fa																
*cc																
Li																
*cc																

Upper

Patient's right side upper jaw   Patient's left side upper jaw

Quadrant No 1   1-1 2-1   Quadrant No 2

1-8   2-8
4-8   3-8

Quadrant No 4   Quadrant No 3

Patient's right side lower jaw   4-1 3-1   Patient's left side lower jaw

Designate implant abutment site in blue

Lower

	4-8	4-7	4-6	4-5	4-4	4-3	4-2	4-1	3-1	3-2	3-3	3-4	3-5	3-6	3-7	3-8
Li																
*cc																
Fa																
*cc																

cate a loose suprastructure. This necessitates a separate procedure in which the attending dentist removes the prosthesis, checks the gold screws for breakage, or determines the need for screw tightening. Mobility of a prosthesis that closely approximates the gingival tissues can only be determined by observing whether the prosthesis rocks when lateral pressure is applied.

Accurate assessment of transmucosal abutment mobility can be performed only if the suprastructure is removed (Fig. 15-3). If movement of the transmucosal abutment is detected, the center abutment screw should be checked for the presence of a fracture. If none is found, a tightening of the center screw by the attending dentist should be all that is required.

Percussive testing of the transmucosal abutment has not been widely used as a peri-implant parameter to date. Clinicians who use percussion find that it is a helpful tool in assessing the presence or absence of sensitivity of the bone surrounding the implant. Under optimal conditions, there should be no bone sensitivity during percussive testing. If sensitivity is found, it should be documented and correlated with other clinical findings.

Of all the clinical parameters used to access the status of the dental implant, assessment of implant mobility and radiographic evaluation of the surrounding bone-implant interface currently remain the traditional modes of evaluation in determining the status of the osseointegrated implant. Radiographs are useful in assessing bone height and density and in showing the functional relationship between the implant, the abutment, and the prosthesis. Although it is a late sign, radiographic evidence of bone loss is the most reliable of all the conventional periodontal indices for evaluating implants. A failing and mobile implant may display a thin radiolucent line at its bone interface.

Panoramic or periapical (perifixtural) baseline radiographs are taken at the time of the abutment connection procedure to ensure that the abutment has been seated properly on the implant. A precise fit between the implant head and the abutment should be evident, with no intervening gap between the two. Perifixtural radiographs are taken subsequent to the seating of the prosthesis. Two views of each

implant are usually required to ensure a more accurate measurement of the marginal bone height around the implant threads. Films are used as a baseline for comparison of bone height with future radiographs. If no film grid is used, bone loss may be assessed by comparing baseline bone height levels and by counting the number of implant threads coronal to the bony crest. With the Nobelpharma implant, the distance between each thread is 0.6 mm. An exact paralleling technique, as well as a standard kilovoltage, will improve radiographic diagnosis.

Protocols for radiographic intervals include baseline films when the prosthesis is seated and follow-up radiographs at 6 months, 1 year, and 3 years after prosthesis insertion. Thereafter, radiographs are taken at 3-year intervals or as needed for necessary evaluation. Many clinicians rely on clinical signs of disease activity (inflammation, mobility, suppuration, recent history of bone loss, etc.) or symptoms, such as pain, sensitivity, or discomfort, to determine the need for additional radiographs.

INSTRUMENTATION

Calculus removal is accomplished by using a plastic scaler to avoid altering the metal surface (Figs. 15-4 to 15-7). Metal instruments, including ultrasonic scalers, are not recommended. Calculus that forms on the transmucosal abutments is primarily supragingival and can be similar to calculus forming on a natural tooth. It will sometimes flake off or easily fracture in large pieces. At other times, the calculus is fine in nature, and its adherence to the abutment cylinder can be tenacious (Fig. 15-8). When it is dried with air, thin calculus may appear burnished, dull, or translucent.

A major goal of transmucosal abutment instrumentation is to avoid roughening the surface. A roughened surface may promote subsequent bacterial plaque accumulation and calculus formation. Additionally, surface alteration of the tin oxide layer has the potential to affect the biologic properties of the surface. Whether a roughened surface has an adverse effect on cell attachment to titanium has not been firmly established in the scientific literature; however, this may be an important consideration.

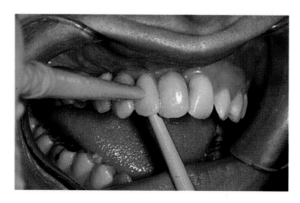

Figure 15-2

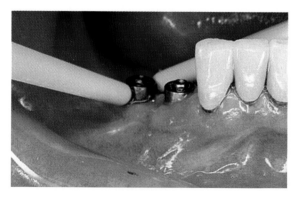

Figure 15-3

After the removal of hard deposits, the prosthesis and transmucosal abutments may be selectively polished with a rubber cup, rubber prophy cup, rubber prophy point, and tufted floss or flossing cord (Figs. 15-9 to 15-11). Aluminum oxide polishing paste is recommended to avoid unnecessary scratching of the titanium abutments and the prosthetic suprastructure. Stains on the suprastructure may require a medium-grit abrasive for complete stain removal.

PATIENT EDUCATION

The long-term success of the dental implant lies, to a great extent, in the ability of the patient to control daily plaque accumulation. The dental professional plays an important role in assisting and influencing the dental patient to maintain an adequate oral hygiene level. The challenge to the dental patient may be one of access because it is often difficult to physically reach all areas of the supragingival appliance despite high levels of motivation. On the other hand, many patients exhibit low dental IQs as evidenced by their denture history. These individuals often require special consideration and patience on the part of the dental professional. More frequent recall intervals may be necessary to encourage compliance. Home care instructions should be reviewed and reinforced at each appointment. Written instructions are

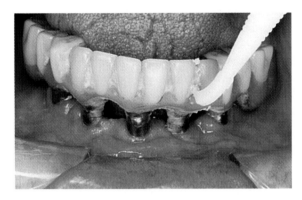

Figure 15-4

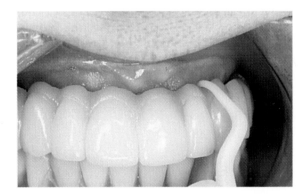

Figure 15-5

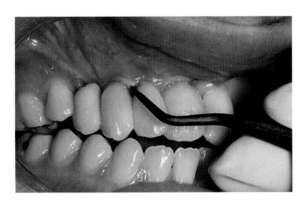

Figure 15-6

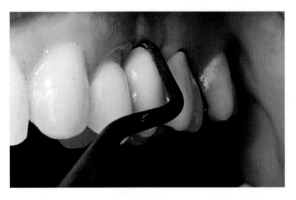

Figure 15-7

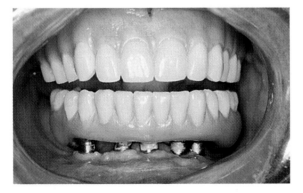

Figure 15-8

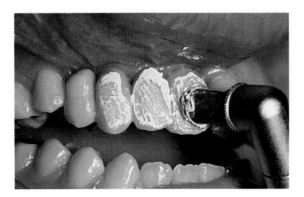

Figure 15-9

often helpful. A variety of cleaning methods may be recommended, depending on the type of design of the prosthesis.

RECOMMENDATIONS AFTER STAGE 2 SURGERY

Absence of microbiota is essential for tissue healing; therefore the presence of plaque will retard the healing process. After the periodontal pack has been removed, plaque forms readily on the abutments.

Initial oral hygiene instructions are given at the time of periodontal pack and suture removal. Recommendations include rinsing with salt water twice a day until the tissue swelling subsides. A twice-daily, 30-second chlorhexidine (Peridex) rinse is recommended for at least 1 week after stage 2 surgery. In some cases rinsing may be continued until the final prosthesis is seated; this is at the clinician's discretion. A soft toothbrush or flat end-tuft brush is used in addition to rinsing (Fig. 15-12). Gentle brushing is important because the patient may experience soft-tissue sensitivity for a period of time after the surgical procedure.

RECOMMENDATIONS FOR COMPLETE AND PARTIALLY EDENTULOUS PATIENTS

An assortment of brushes may be used to effectively remove soft deposits. A standard toothbrush is usually recommended for the facial, lingual, and occlusal surfaces of the prosthetic suprastructure. A nylon-coated interdental brush is effective for plaque removal on the gingival side of the suprastructure and proximal surfaces of the abutments. A flat end-tuft brush is indicated on the facial surfaces of the abutment cylinders. This brush is angled 45 degrees toward the gingival tissues and moved in a circular, vibratory motion. The tapered end-tuft brush is preferred for plaque removal on lingual abutment surfaces. The brush head may be bent to improve access to this area (Fig. 15-13).

Prosthetic bridge design and patient dexterity dictate selection of the type of floss or flossing cord. A flossing cord specifically designed for dental implants polishes the transmucosal abutments and the gingival side of the prosthesis. The hooked end of the cord is used as a threading device,

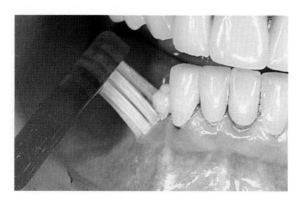

Figure 15-10

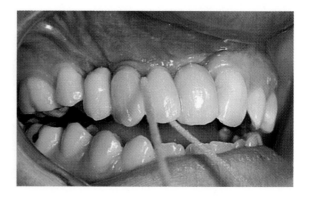

Figure 15-11

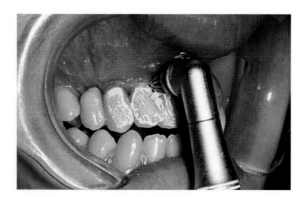

Figure 15-12

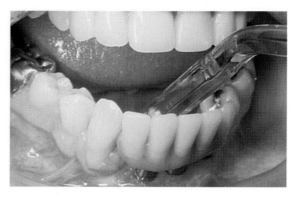

Figure 15-13

making insertion between adjacent abutment cylinders relatively easy (Fig. 15-14). Once inserted, the cord is criss-crossed and moved from side to side and up and down to reach the entire circumference of the abutment (Fig. 15-15). A thinner cord for light embrasures may be used; the cord is durable enough to be used several times by simply rinsing and drying after each use.

Rotary brushes may be a helpful adjunct to the home care regimen. Caution should be taken in areas of nonkeratinized tissue or implant thread exposure (Fig. 15-16).

RECOMMENDATIONS FOR SINGLE-TOOTH PROSTHESIS

Home care recommendations for cleaning the single-tooth implant prosthesis vary depending on the prosthetic and abutment design and on its location in the mouth. A soft toothbrush is recommended for brushing the crown and prosthetic components surrounded by the gingiva. If the transmucosal abutment is placed subgingivally, regular dental floss or tufted floss may be used. The prosthetic tooth is flossed in the same manner as a natural tooth, wrapping the floss around the narrow circumference of the abutment cylinder (Fig. 15-17). Nylon-coated interdental brushes are helpful in cleaning the proximal surfaces. The appropriate brush size is determined by the space available, which varies from patient to patient.

RECOMMENDATIONS FOR OVERDENTURE PROSTHESIS

Home care for the patient with an overdenture is facilitated by removing the overdenture. The transmucosal abutments may be brushed with either a standard soft toothbrush or a flat end-tuft brush (Fig. 15-18). If the abutment cylinders are connected with a bar, floss or a flossing cord is easily inserted under the bar and then wrapped around each abutment cylinder for cleaning (Fig. 15-19).

Cleaning the undersurface of the prosthesis, the overdenture framework, and the proximal surfaces of the abutment cylinders may be accomplished using a nylon-coated interdental brush (Fig. 15-20). Patients should be encouraged to

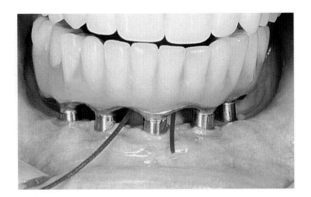

Figure 15-14

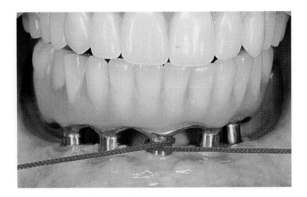

Figure 15-15

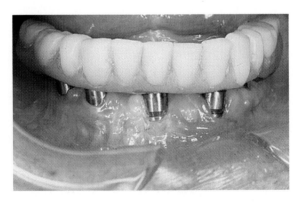

Figure 15-16

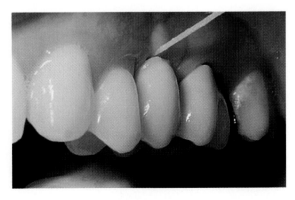

Figure 15-17

replace the interdental brushes frequently because the underlying metal wire, if exposed, may scratch the titanium surface.

A daily soaking of the overdenture in a commercial cleaning solution is recommended. If no metal is present on the prosthesis, an overnight soaking in full-strength white vinegar once each week is helpful in removing stubborn stains.

At the clinician's discretion, other adjunctive oral hygiene aids, such as rubber tips and wooden picks, may be recommended. A toothpaste accepted by the American Dental Association may be used during brushing. Twice-daily antimicrobial rinses, such as chlorhexidine, may be beneficial if patients are unable to maintain adequate oral hygiene levels. These individuals should be informed of possible side effects, such as staining and taste alteration. Altered taste may be minimized by using the rinse at least 1 hour after food consumption.

Subgingival oral irrigation may be a helpful adjunct for selected patients. Caution must be taken to adjust the rate of flow to the lowest setting. The patient is instructed to direct the antimicrobial solution into the sulcus, allowing the solution to gently flood the sulcus.

Other home care recommendations and instructions are influenced by the location, angulation, and length of the transmucosal abutments; the prosthetic design; and the patient's oral habits, motivation, manual dexterity, and oral health. Careful, individualized instruction is usually required with any dental implant patient.

MAINTENANCE INTERVALS

Maintenance intervals are determined by several factors, such as the amount of plaque and calculus formation, the condition of the soft tissues, the status of the prosthesis, the patient's commitment to meticulous home care, and various health considerations of the patient. Appropriate recall intervals are determined on an individual basis, taking into consideration the patient's history and present evaluation. A suggested time frame may be the following:

1. At prosthesis delivery
   - Comprehensive oral hygiene instructions
   - Baseline data documented
2. One month after prosthesis delivery
   - Review of home care techniques
   - Calculus removal and coronal polish, if needed
3. Three months later
   - Examination of tissues
   - Calculus removal and coronal polish, if needed
   - Home care reinforcement
   - Establishment of a recall interval (between 3 and 6 months, determined by history and current assessment)

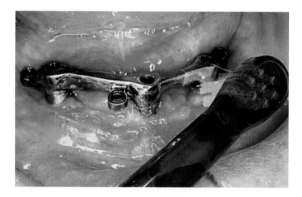

Figure 15-18

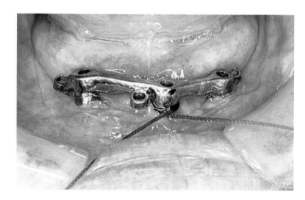

Figure 15-19

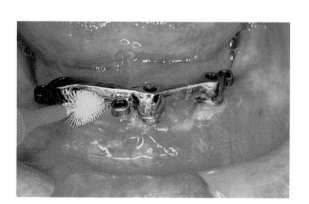

Figure 15-20

INDEX

Page numbers in *italics* indicate illustrations.